HOW I GREW YOUNGER

And Why You Should Too...

In just 2 weeks, you can reduce belly fat, cholesterol, inflammation, and the age of your arteries with the BalancePoint diet

BINX SELBY
LINDA JADE FONG

Necton Press

This book is intended to be informational and should not be considered a substitute for advice from a medical professional (see "A Message to the Reader" before the Introduction of this book).

Mention of specific companies, organizations, or authorities in this book does not imply endorsement by the authors or publisher, nor does mention of specific companies, organizations, or authorities imply that they endorse this book, its authors, or the publisher.

ISBN 978-1481159241

First edition
Designed by Gustavo Estrella
of
rollick
CREATIVE

Necton Press

Necton Press
PO Box 6006
Boulder, Colorado 80306

We wish that we had known what we do now about reducing inflammation when our fathers, Howard Selby and John Fong, died from stroke disease and cancer.

We dedicate this book to their memories and to our mothers, Marian Tofel and Hazel Fong, who have always nurtured the explorer in us.

ACKNOWLEDGMENTS

When a book has been over six years in the making, there are a lot of people whose direct or indirect contribution has been much appreciated. This is a partial list, with apologies to those we have inadvertently missed:

- **Robert Kerr**, for constant and invaluable involvement on both a professional and personal level with the BalancePoint protocol;
- **Michael Weitekamp, M.D.** of Penn State Hershey for presenting our results to the American College of Cardiology, and **Stephen Archer, M.D.** of the University of Chicago, and two former presidents of the American Heart Association, **Joseph Alpert, M.D.** of the University of Arizona, and **Robert Eckel, M.D.** of the University of Colorado, for opportunities to present my data to them;
- **Shelley Schlender**, for contributions to this book, indefatigable brainstorming sessions, and networking for me to show my early results to researchers including **Loren Cordane, Ph.D., Ron Rosedale, M.D., Richard Feinman, Ph.D., Stephen Phinney, M.D., PhD**.
- **Richard Williams, Ph.D., John O'Hearne, M.D., Robert Selby, M.D.,** and **Robert Kerr, J.D.** for co-authoring with me the medical paper, *"Dietary protocol for a rapid reduction of risk levels of cholesterols, triglycerides, and arterial stiffness: a before/after study of a pilot dietary program."*
- **James Ehrlich, M.D., Gary Kahn, M.D., David Mendosa, Mort Rosenblum, Jerry Sears, Ellen Sears** and **Sandra Mihalko** for advice and networking;
- **Dianne Schroeder** and **Caitlin Cegavske** for suggestions and close reading of the final draft and **James, Cynthia, Diane, Glenn, Daniela, Bonnie,** and **Jane** for earlier proofing and critiques;
- **Kathy, Kevin, Colleen, Lizi, Joan,** and **Stephanie** for working directly with BalancePoint participants over the years to help them get best results from the protocol.
- **Gustavo Estrella** for the intelligent and beautiful design of this book
- Our daughter, **Linx Selby**, for designing the logo and coming up with this book's title when she found ours "too boring", and for contributing feedback, photos and creative BalancePoint dishes as she scrupulously follows the protocol and explains the benefits to others, whether it is to friends seeking clear complexions or university staff wanting to prevent strokes.
- All the BalancePoint participants for sharing their own motivations, experiences, data, and recipes, and especially the Trident Coffee Shop gang for becoming the first set of guinea pigs so many years ago and then pressing for the completion of this book ever since.

To all, and to many more unnamed here, we are grateful.

TABLE OF CONTENTS

A MESSAGE TO THE READER

The information in this book is designed to help you make informed choices. It is not intended to substitute for expert medical advice or treatment. This book contains the opinions and ideas of the authors, who are not doctors or medical practitioners. The advice and strategies contained in this book may not be suitable for your situation; you should consult with a professional. Because each individual is unique, a physician or other health care practitioner must diagnose conditions and supervise treatments for each individual health problem, and this professional guidance should be followed if contrary to information provided in this book.

While the authors and publisher have used their best efforts in preparing this book, they make no representations or warranties with respect to the accuracy or completeness of the contents of this book or fitness for a particular purpose. They specifically disclaim all responsibility for any liability, loss, or risk, personal or otherwise, which may be incurred as a consequence, directly or indirectly, of the use and application of any of the contents of this book.

INTRODUCTION

It happened within days—arteries measuring 30 years younger

I *asked Dr. Ehrlich, "Do you often get readings like this?"* It was by accident that I discovered how we could turn back the clock on the age of our arteries.

Your arteries may be stiff, and may have aged faster than your chronological age, and you may not even know it. You will likely not be aware of it, either, until an out-of-the-blue stroke or serious heart problem occurs. The good news is that you do not have to wait to find out the hard way. You can bring back elasticity to your arteries and overall health to your body through the food you eat.

In 2006, I created a new diet that was getting remarkable results in balancing people's cholesterol levels in only two weeks. I took my data to the president of the American Heart Association in Denver.

After the meeting, we stopped by Dr. James Ehrlich's heart imaging clinic. I wanted to show my brother Robert, a professor of medicine at the University of Arizona, a machine I intended to use in my research. It was an instrument found mainly in medical research labs to measure the elasticity of arteries—a direct indicator of risk level for stroke or related heart problems.

Dr. Ehrlich connected Robert to the slightly-smaller-than-a-breadbox device and the results were not surprising. Robert was riding 150 miles a week on his bike and conscientiously eating a Mediterranean—not my new—diet. Graphs flashed up on the computer screen showing the strong heart capacity of an athlete and a level of stiffness in the arteries like that of someone a few years younger than his age.

Clearly pleased, Robert then rushed out the door for the airport. We too got ready to leave, when a man in his 60's from our group asked if he could get tested too. He had started my diet a couple months earlier with a size 40 waist. He had used the diet to lower his cholesterol. He was still on the protocol and had a goal—which he later made--of fitting back into his size 34 cashmere pants.

Dr. Ehrlich kept re-positioning the sensor on the man's wrist and re-taking readings. I looked at the graphs and said, "You're getting a good waveform, why do you keep re-doing it?" The doctor looked at his portly subject and dubiously asked, "Are you in really good shape?" His arterial health was measuring like that of a 35-year-old—not what the doctor was expecting.

It hit me. "It's the diet! It's the diet!" I shouted excitedly.

I turned to my wife. "Try Linda! She's been on the diet too. Let's see how she comes out." Well, her arteries came out to be the equivalent of a 32-year-old, which was 20 years younger than her age. Next was me, who had been on the diet for the longest time, about six months at this point. I had actually been measured a few weeks earlier and once again my reading came out to be like a 29-year-old, over 30 years younger than my age. This time, though, I was seeing others measuring "young."

I asked Dr. Ehrlich, "Do you often get readings like this?" "No," he answered. "Let me show you," and he put the sensor on his own wrist.

His face went white. The graph of his "internal blood pressure" printed a lot of red bars and showed his vascular age equivalency to be that of a 75-year-old. He was actually in his early 50's. "No doctor would prescribe anything for me because my cuff blood pressure is normal," he muttered.

Instead, Dr. Ehrlich came up to our office in Boulder to find out how to do my protocol. The next week my cell phone rang as we were driving through the Rockies to pick up our daughter from summer violin camp. "Binx, I'm on the third day of your diet," he exclaimed. "And since the Sphygmocor was sitting right there in my office I thought I'd do another reading. It's already gone down 30 years! In a couple of days!"

The speed of change was my first clue that it was probably inflammation that we were reducing.

It's now been six years since that visit to Dr. Ehrlich's clinic. The protocol, which has come to be known as BalancePoint, has remained the same. Both my wife and I have seen our arterial age equivalency go down to the level of a teenager's, and we've seen some peoples' get reduced by six decades. In a study *(See Appendix 1)*, the average reduction was almost 20 years.

The food protocol that I am going to share with you will decrease the chronic inflammation level in your body. Chronic inflammation lies at the root of most age-related diseases and the newest medical literature keeps adding to the list: stroke and heart disease, belly fat, osteoarthritis, Type II diabetes, hypertension, periodontal disease, certain autoimmune diseases, many types of cancer, Alzheimer's, micro-stroke dementia.

So it is not only your arteries which could experience a rapid rejuvenation. This book will show you what else and explain why.

Binx Selby
Boulder, Colorado 2012

This book is Binx's story. As a scientist, he has a passion for research and data as well as an enthusiastic desire to share his knowledge. The sharing is where I come in. I've gathered and absorbed a myriad of notes and presentations over the past six years as Binx and I have guided hundreds of people through the BalancePoint protocol. This book is the outcome—an offering to you, the reader, to review the data and results, ponder the theories, delight in the anecdotes and recipes, and try this revolutionary program which can bring about significant health improvements in only days. Binx's motto is, "Heart disease may very well be optional," and his mission is to show how you can take control of your health in ways you never realized were possible. We invite you to give it a go!

Linda Jade Fong

PART ONE

Heart disease may very well be optional

***BalancePoint:** A breakthrough food protocol that quickly reduces inflammation in your body to make your arteries younger and bring your cardiovascular and metabolic systems to optimal health*

"A man is as old as his arteries."

THOMAS SYDENHAM, "THE ENGLISH HIPPOCRATES," 1624-89

Do you know how old your arteries are? This 400-year-old wisdom from "The Father of English Medicine" is being rediscovered today as we find many people whose blood vessels have aged beyond their years. Our research has shown that many people have arteries that are like those of someone 20, 30, even 40 or 50 years older. Even young people and athletes can have surprisingly stiff arteries that put them at high risk for strokes and heart disease.

I want to share with you a way of eating ordinary food that can make your arteries measure decades younger.

This protocol also works better than drugs to drop cholesterol.

Plus, you get the bonus of losing weight and belly fat in a healthy way and without feeling like you're starving.

You can see these results in **less than two weeks**.

Better yet, the results are backed by medical data.

It sounds almost too good to be true to get such significant results so rapidly. The reason is the strong anti-inflammatory power of this diet. Inflammation is now known to be a root cause of most aging-related diseases and imbalances in our cardiovascular and metabolic systems.

Take a look at these major benefits of the BalancePoint diet that have been drawing the attention of doctors and cardiologists:

1. Reduction of the age-equivalency of one's arteries by an average of 20 years. The stiffness of your arteries can be tested with a medical research instrument using a technique called sphygmography. It gives a direct measurement of how flexible your arteries are, and you can readily see the result of reversing inflammation in your arteries. The measurements are compared to normal arteries for different ages on an FDA-approved database. On this chart, the arteries of both my co-author and myself show the elasticity found in teenagers.

2. Fast, dramatic cholesterol changes - When we talk about "high cholesterol", people often make the mistake of looking at their "total cholesterol" number. That is a misleading number and we will teach you how to look at cholesterol numbers with the benefit of the newest knowledge. But, before we get to that, you should know that cholesterol results typically show a breakdown between what is known as the "bad" LDL cholesterol and the "good" HDL cholesterol.

2-WEEK BALANCEPOINT RESULTS

fig. 1

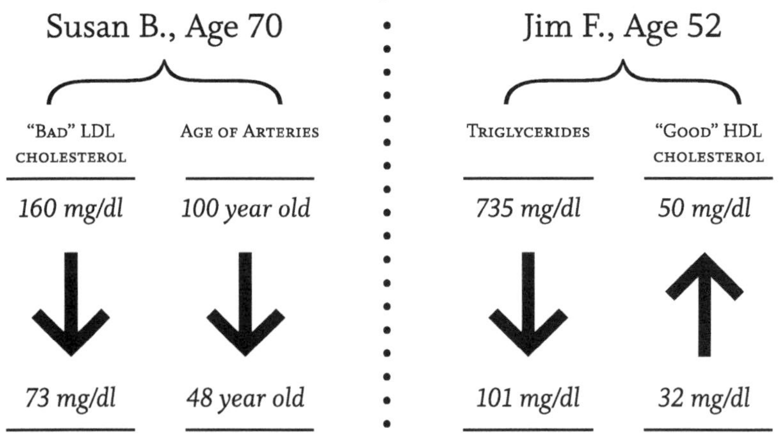

**In contrast to BalancePoint, statin drugs have not been shown to decrease the stiffness or age of arteries, nor decrease triglycerides, nor increase HDLs*

Doctors like to see levels of LDL "bad" cholesterol close to or below 100 mg/dl. We have medical results to show how 70-year-old Susan B. dropped her LDL cholesterol from 160 to 73. That is a drop of 87 points in two weeks on BalancePoint. In addition, her arteries, which measured as stiff as a 100-year-old's before BalancePoint, regained the flexibility of a 45-year-old in these same fourteen days.

In another case, 52-year-old Jim F. saw his triglycerides plummet from a very high 735 to an optimal level of 101 mg/dl and his "good" HDLs rise 45%, again in two weeks. These two examples drawn out of hundreds of BalancePoint medically-monitored results demonstrate this ground-breaking research and development.

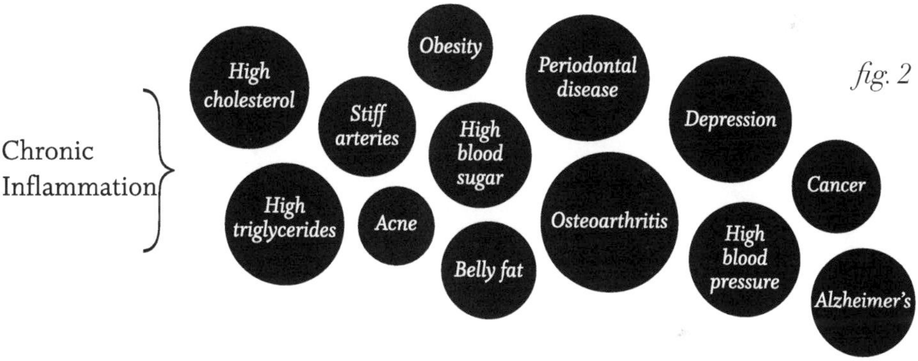

Chronic inflammation has been increasingly linked to a wide range of diseases.

3. Bringing cholesterol and cardiovascular conditions to optimal health in a very short time is an expected outcome of the BalancePoint protocol.

We presented BalancePoint data at the American College of Cardiology 2009 Annual Meeting to compare our cholesterol results *to a New England Journal of Medicine* study of the three most popular diets in the country right now. As you can see from the chart (fig.3) in this chapter, the most that either a low-fat, Mediterranean or low-carb diet did in reducing what is called the "bad" LDL cholesterol was a decrease of 5.6 mg/dl in six months.

In comparison, **the BalancePoint diet showed an average LDL cholesterol drop of 52.1 mg/dl. That is almost 10 times greater.** And this was accomplished in two weeks.

4. Even though we are told to decrease the level of LDL cholesterol,

Cardiovascular disease, or disease of the heart and arteries, is the major cause of death in the Western world. Pick two of your best friends, and all three of you stand in front of a mirror. Look into the mirror—statistics say one of you has cardiovascular disease. Coronary artery disease is the leading cause of most forms of cardiovascular disease, such as strokes and heart problems. It can begin in childhood and is usually not detectable. The first symptom is often a heart attack or, in up to one-third of patients, sudden death. ***BalancePoint can reverse the inflammation that causes coronary artery disease and other conditions also related to inflammation in the body. The reversal happens quickly and without drugs.***

medical researchers will tell you that not all LDLs are equal. That is why cardiologists will refer patients with cardiovascular risk to a test which calculates the proportion of "small particle size" LDLs, which are the most dangerous form, versus "large, buoyant" LDLs, which are actually needed by the body for cell repair. We frequently see people's LDL profiles change after going on the BalancePoint diet to show a bigger proportion of large buoyant LDLs versus the small, dense ones, which can infiltrate cell walls to cause damage.

Unlike results from BalancePoint, statin drugs lower all LDLs, including the beneficial ones and not just the specific problematic ones. Also, statins do not generally lower triglycerides or raise HDLs.

5. Some people also use the BalancePoint diet to **lose weight.** It may be to get rid of belly fat, which is very difficult to do on regular diets even using exercise, but which BalancePoint appears to target. Or, it may be to lose 15 pounds to fit better into an old pair of cashmere pants or 65 plus pounds (the record we are aware of is over 140 pounds) to regain health. The average weight drop in two weeks is eight pounds (*See Appendix 1*).

6. And, while people find they can lose pounds easily with BalancePoint, **you do not have to lose weight to get these same spectacular cholesterol drops**.

If you do choose to go for weight reduction through BalancePoint, your new lower cholesterol level stays the same even after your weight stabilizes. This is a point especially for doctors to note. They see patients lower their cholesterol numbers as long as they are losing weight, but those numbers go back up once you stop losing weight. Not so with BalancePoint.

We get the satisfaction of seeing results like those in fig. 4 consistently come in to us. There is a special kick out of having someone send in a copy of his blood test results with hand-scribbled doctor's comments, like "WOW!"

We have found that the BalancePoint protocol works for about 95% of the people who are able to strictly follow the protocol and use a nutritional tracker to ensure exact compliance.

Other anti-inflammatory benefits of BalancePoint

As if the cholesterol improvement were not enough, BalancePoint diet participants report other welcome changes. We have had over 400 people on the BalancePoint diet in the last six years and here are some of the non-cholesterol benefits they have noted:

- **Weight control**, whether it is loss, maintenance or gain that you want
- **Decrease of arthritic pain**
- **Decrease of allergies**
- **Improvement of blood sugar levels**
- **Improvement of skin conditions** such as acne and rosacea

At first glance, the range of these benefits of the BalancePoint diet may seem hard to believe for many people. But if you are someone who likes to keep up with leading edge medical research, it will become clear to you why all these effects are possible. It is now accepted medical belief that heart disease and strokes and, in fact, almost all chronic health conditions related to aging are being traced to inflammation in the body. This belief for many medical researchers extends to including Alzheimer's and some cancers in this group of diseases. In the past couple of years we have seen an explosion of medical studies looking at how chronic inflammation is a common source of different ailments related to our cardiovascular and metabolic systems. These include high cholesterol, stiffening of the arteries, high blood pressure, obesity, and type-2 diabetes.

It takes only days to notice the effect. How many other things have you done in your life that can prove themselves so quickly?

This is where the revolutionary approach of BalancePoint comes in. In short, the BalancePoint diet is scientifically designed to act at the level of the metabolic pathways of the body—at the root of the problem. Not only does it act at this very basic source level. It also has a significant anti-inflammatory effect. You will see in a later chapter how we believe this diet creates an environment in the body which allows it to heal itself. So, instead of producing an inflammatory response which triggers and manifests itself in a variety of conditions, the body begins its own repair... naturally.

You do not have to take our word for it. You can look at our medical data, such as blood tests collected at independent hospital labs. You can read our analysis. Or, even better, you can simply try the BalancePoint protocol yourself. It takes only days to notice the effect. How many other things have you done in your life that can prove themselves so quickly? If aggressive lifestyle change is something you feel you have the discipline and motivation to try instead of taking drugs, then read further!

What makes up the diet?

So what is the diet? The food is common, everyday food you would find on grocery shelves. However, there are specific types and exact amounts of this food that we prescribe for you on a daily basis.

Basically, **BalancePoint is a precise formula of foods**. It is strictly defined because it is designed to act in a particular biochemical way. This formula is made up of very carefully calculated proportions of high-fat content (healthy fats like olive oil, nuts and avocados), low Glycemic-index carbohydrates (such as found in leafy greens and most kinds of fresh fruit rather than the high-Glycemic carbs in foods like grains), and low protein (such as egg whites, strained Greek-style yogurt, and tofu during the first two weeks and then managed amounts of fish, chicken and grass-fed red meat later). The total calorie level is limited. You will read throughout the book the reasons for the choice and amounts of these foods. There are no special supplements, only fish oil tablets, regular multivitamins, and psyllium fiber. Coffee and tea, as well as wine and cocoa are allowed—an added attraction for many!

You will not feel hungry like on a typical diet and you will be delighted by delicious tastes, both due to the high oil content and the use of a variety of spices.

You will have your work cut out for you, however, during the two-week education phase. Since this is a formula, you will have to measure and track all the food you eat during our two-week Jumpstart program to ensure that

> *Our food should be our medicine. Our medicine should be our food."*
>
> - Hippocrates

you are within the formula. To do this you need to accurately follow the instructions and develop a sense of this new way of eating.

This is not like a typical weight-loss diet which gives you general guidelines to follow. We actually refer to it as a ***protocol***, because it is an exact food formula that is scientifically engineered to act with the same precision of a drug on our metabolic system. Think of it as a prescription, but one which uses delicious, everyday foods instead of drugs.

If you and your doctor decide this is the approach you want to try, you must understand that it is a lifestyle change. The two-week BalancePoint Jumpstart is to train you and get you going on a healthy track for the rest of your life. The American Medical Association recommends that doctors try prescribing lifestyle changes before drugs for lowering cholesterol, so BalancePoint is for those people motivated to try this option.

We have found that if you are totally compliant with the protocol, you stand a good chance of getting the results we talk about. That means no guessing, no estimating, no changing, no adapting the protocol. No cheating! If you are short even as little as 1 ½ tablespoons of oil each day you will get only half the results you should be able to achieve. They will most likely be results which will still impress your doctor, but will not be in the jaw-dropping range which you are probably capable of achieving.

Part V of this book will give you a how-to on doing the diet yourself. We will teach you how you can use common food, the kind you would find in your local supermarket, in precisely measured portions to fit our formula for success. We will also show you how to prepare them in tasty, satisfying ways so that you will not feel the normal hunger pangs associated with diets. For some of you, this how-to section may be all you want out of the book at this time.

BalancePoint's revolutionary concepts

However, for those who are curious and intrigued about the scientific basis of this diet, you will also find in this book some of the **ground-breaking medical concepts and discoveries that BalancePoint offers**, including my theories about the links between inflammation, cholesterol and lipid metabolism:

- **Very high fat diet** – Why and how I came to defy the conventional mantra of "low fat" to design a high fat diet to *"fight fat with fat"* and reduce belly fat and cholesterol
- **Activation of fat-burning mode** – My discovery of the importance—and mechanism—to ***turn on, and keep running, our lipid metabolism, instead of our usual fat-storing carbohydrate metabolism***

Fight fat with fat

- **Specific food protocol** – How the BalancePoint diet resets our body's metabolic pathways with an extremely precise, patent-pending dietary formula that is engineered to act in the body with the same precision as a drug
- **Breakthrough results** – How our protocol produces repeatable and reproducible results unheard of in the medical world for speed of non-drug cholesterol reduction and effectiveness that goes beyond drugs
- **A technique that works** – How BalancePoint has gone beyond theory to offer a clinical application and actual data to support elements of the diet which are now appearing as theory in the medical literature
- **Role of inflammation** – My theory on how inflammation is the cause and not the effect of high cholesterol and other medical conditions. I suspect it is inflammation—that which is underlying the cholesterol and plaque build-up in our arteries—which is the true culprit
- **Cause of inflammation** – As an extension of the above theory, I believe that it is diet, not cholesterol, which is the primary cause of inflammation, and therefore heart disease, in the arteries
- **Anti-inflammatory properties of the diet give significant cardiovascular and metabolic improvements** – How the BalancePoint protocol provides an environment in which the body can heal itself, and

so can result in considerable progress in treating inflammatory-related conditions, ranging from stiffening of the arteries and osteoarthritis to high glucose levels and obesity

I continue to be surprised at ***how quickly the body can take over and repair itself.*** Before BalancePoint, we all thought it was a slow process to lower cholesterol without drugs. Six years later, the hundreds of people who have followed our two-week Jumpstart protocol show how fast it can happen.

As you read this book, you will learn how and why the BalancePoint diet **improves health** in many of the ways described above. But for most people, it all starts by seeking a solution to one of the most urgent issues many of us face these days—a cardiovascular or metabolic problem. High cholesterol is a prime example.

In fact, that is how it happened with me...

A Facebook comment from a newspaper editor:

Wayne L. Speaking of Linda, she and her husband Binx developed an amazing eating/lifestyle program that they originally invented as a way to control cholesterol - which it did. I went on it for about a year and wound up in the best shape of my life. At age 42, a cardiologist told me I had the circulatory elasticity of a teenager. I lost about 80 pounds and ran a 50-minute 10K Bolder Boulder. Unfortunately, I have gone astray. I must return to the BalancePoint program.

20 minutes ago · Like

COMPARISON OF DIETS FOR LOWERING LDL CHOLESTEROL

fig. 3

BalancePoint data presented at American College of Cardiology Annual Meeting, March 2009

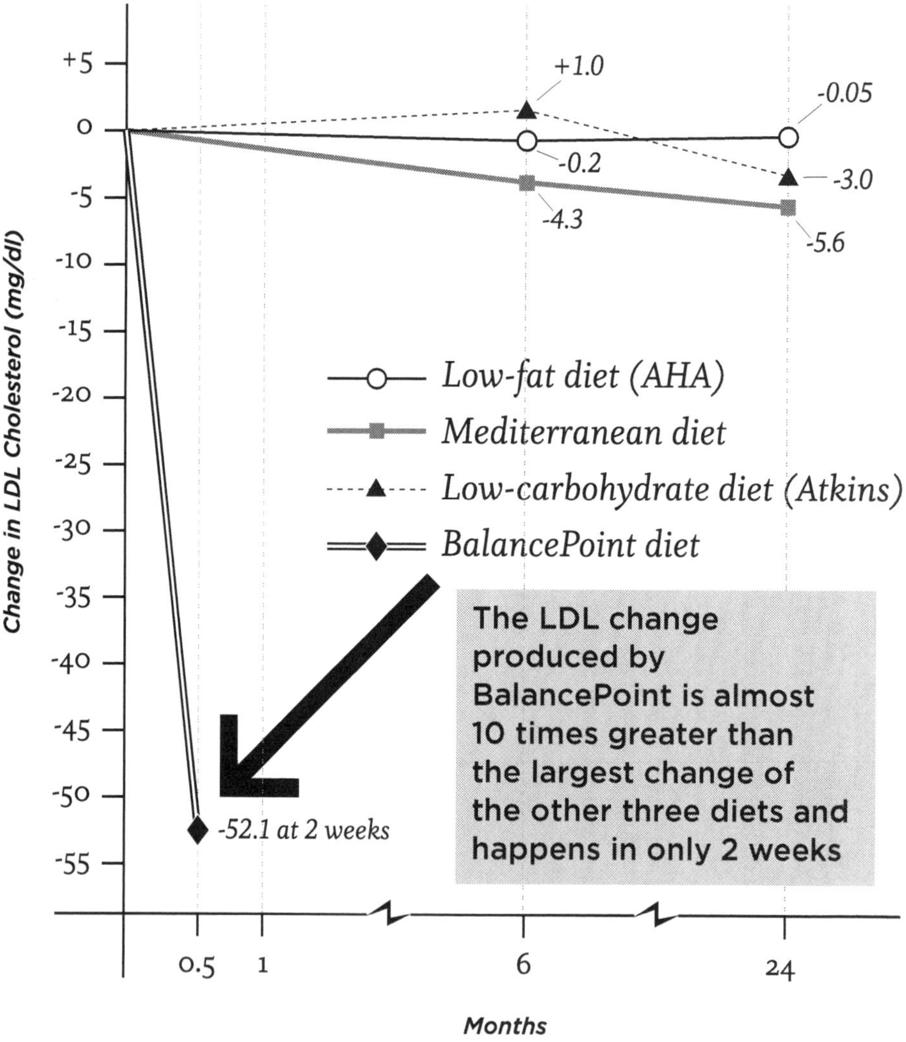

Data for the American Heart Association, Mediterranean, and Atkins diets is from the DIRECT Study [Shai I., et al. Weight Loss with Low-Carbohydrate, Mediterranean, or Low-Fat Diet. *N Engl J Med* 2008: 359:229-241, Figure 3 Page 239.]

PART TWO

Crisis as Opportunity

How Binx discovered the BalancePoint solution

"Heart disease may very well be optional"

- Binx Selby

CHAPTER 1

Urgent Inspiration: The Two-Week Medical Challenge

The crisis

危机

The Chinese character for "crisis" is made up of two parts: "danger" and "opportunity"

It all started back at the end of the year 2005 when my thumb turned purple.

Not only was it a dark purple, it was cold and hard to the touch. After two days, fearing my thumb might wither away and fall off, I walked into the rural clinic where I was vacationing to get it checked.

The physician on duty looked at my thumb and decided to put in a phone call to a vascular specialist for advice. I waited about two and a half hours, and then she returned with a syringe in one hand and directions to the closest big city emergency ward in the other.

"This could be serious," she said.

In the syringe was blood thinner, and I knew there was concern about possible arterial blockage. So when I returned back home a couple days later, I scurried over to my longtime family doctor, a highly competent and respected physician who was adept at putting up with my tendency to question everything. She attributed the purple thumb to Raynaud's Syndrome, a relatively harmless condition in which fingers or toes become purple in response to cold or stress (and which I did not know at the time ran in my family).

Just to be safe, though, the doctor ordered a test called a calcium scan, which looks at the blood vessels feeding the heart. Evidence indicates that the more calcification you have, the greater the potential for heart disease.

Well, my numbers came out high—deep into the high-risk area.

At that time, my total cholesterol was 219, my HDL "good" cholesterol was 80 mg/dl and my LDL "bad" cholesterol was 117. (Doctors like to see HDL levels above 60 and LDL levels below 129.) Under normal circumstances these levels would be considered fine.

Not in this case, though. My doctor told me, "With this calcium score, we need to get your LDLs way down under 100. *Right away.*

"So I'm going to put you on statins."

Statins are a category of very effective cholesterol-lowering drugs which have saved countless lives by preventing the heart attacks and strokes associated with high cholesterol. Statins are the most widely prescribed drugs in the world, in fact. But they are not without side effects. For example, users need an annual test to detect for potential liver problems that can be caused by the drugs.

"Isn't that a drug I'd have to take for the rest of my life?" I asked.

She nodded.

The opportunity

Then I thought, hold on a minute. I was in my 60's and had just bicycled 40 miles in the Colorado foothills that morning. I beat everyone on the ride, and I felt great. (I liked to tell everyone that I had to bike every day to be able to keep up with my middle-schooler.) I meditated every morning. I was eating what was considered a healthy Mediterranean diet, with lots of vegetables, fruit, grains, cheese, yogurt, and fish. But now my doctor was telling me that I needed a life-long prescription for statins?

Something was wrong with this picture. The body is a piece of incredible natural engineering. In most cases, it is designed to operate without having to take drugs every day.

"No problem can be solved from the same level of consciousness that created it."

- Albert Einstein

Then suddenly I knew I had the answer somewhere in my subconscious. I had a flash that there had to be a nutritional solution to this. In fact, I think it was at this same moment that I had an instant flashback to the metabolic pathways chart that hung on my bedside wall back in graduate school days. This is a chart that basically maps the biochemistry of our bodies. At the time, I did not know why the chart zoomed into my consciousness, but I sensed there was a clue in it for me.

I told my doctor I wanted a little time to work on this problem another way. She gave me two weeks.

Even before reaching my car, I had begun designing in my head a fast way to reduce my cholesterol—without drugs.

No to the prescription pad

The Inventor's Response

I am enjoying my weight loss a lot. But my return to health is even more appreciated!

- Sara C.

Kick-started by the urgency of the situation, I found myself returning to familiar territory—Inventor Mode.

As an inventor with a background in biochemistry and technology, I found my dilemma frightening, yet at the same time fascinating.

I have always found myself trying to solve problems with new solutions. When my two-finger typing resulted in pages stiff with white-out, I devised the first standalone word processing machine, which spawned a large company called NBI and became a leading prototype for the personal computer. Then, after well water at my home in the Colorado mountains came out full of soda, I designed a room-sized, microprocessor-controlled "appliance" named PureCycle which recycled and turned all household water (including medicine-contaminated or... sewage!) into pure drinking water. (I cannot resist noting that the sign above our drinking fountain said, "All water has been passed by Management.") The purification technology is used on the Space Shuttle and also being used for pharmaceutical and computer chip manufacturing processes which require ultrapure water with no detectable traces of contaminants. Another technology I invented was the data storage use of the laser disk which predated CDs and the Internet, and which related to my early ambition to put the Library of Congress in the hands of anyone who wanted it. One other example of a personally motivated invention came out of my first bike trips through Italy. I returned with cravings for their coffee, so in the pre-Starbucks 1990s, I invented an automated espresso machine to reproduce the skills of the best Italian baristas.

Now, after creating more than a dozen products and companies like these which were a response to a personal interest or problem, I faced a new challenge. I needed to fix my cholesterol levels—and fast. My body should be able to repair itself, I reasoned. It just needed the right environment or stimulus. Or nourishing...

Unraveling the pack rat's nest

An outside-the-box approach

Driving home from the doctor's office, my head started pulsating with images and ideas. I want to take you along on this mind tour for several reasons. For one, you will see the clues and thinking that give the diet its scientific basis and success. You will hear why I could embark on something so controversial as eating lots of fat. You will also understand how a non-doctor could come up with a way to dramatically reduce cholesterol without drugs. Lastly, it has been an adventure of discovery, and you might enjoy the ride.

Let me begin by explaining that there are different types of thinking when it comes to problem-solving. For most people, it is a process involving logic. That means methodically reviewing all the medical research first and then coming up with a deduction. Almost everyone assumes that was how this diet came into being. But that was not the way it happened.

It has been fascinating to me how even after telling people otherwise, I often hear them re-tell the story of my discovery as one where I studied the literature and then came up with a new answer. The need to put things into comfortable categories and sequences is deeply ingrained in most people's consciousness. It is a reflex to attach a system or linear pattern to make sense of something.

I honestly do not think I could have come up with the BalancePoint solution, though, if I had done it that way. It would not have lent itself to thinking "outside the box."

I instead often find myself using another kind of thinking, one that is more open-ended and more integrative. Seemingly opposing ideas are not viewed as contradictions. Everything does not need to make sense.

It is also more intuitive. Much like how a child might think, it has been described as "wisdom mind" rather than "rationale mind." It is the type of clear intuition that we might suddenly find when we are in a moment of panic, when there's no time to "think".

You will remember that I did have my moment of panic.

The alarm also had a strange calm accompanying it. In that instant, I felt that the solution to my cholesterol reduction problem was inside me somewhere, waiting to be discovered.

I decided not to do any research, or read any materials, or talk to anyone, beforehand. I have found that avoiding preconceived notions of what is the "right" way—or, conversely, why something can't be done—is useful in the preliminary phase of inventing. This allows a new or different approach, what we call the "outside-the-box" idea, to come forth. This is particularly true in technical areas which are very complex and not always well understood, such as medicine.

Also, as an inventor, I did not want to inject new information that might stop the flow of consciousness.

Picture this flow of images and thoughts about cholesterol and metabolism quickly unraveling from a pack rat's nest—my mind. An inventor relishes collecting every possible bit of information from different sources and disciplines. And, in my case, none of it ever gets thrown out! This could range from technical data and research reports from the latest scientific journals or lectures to anecdotal experiences of fellow bike riders and chorale singers.

In inventor mode, all these seemingly random and unrelated "info-bits" merge into a sort of hologram of knowledge in my mind. The hologram has no precisely defined components or structure, just a vague vision. Its formlessness is the kind of thing that drives most people crazy. As I explained earlier, it is not a linear path, like a methodical survey or analysis of the literature leading to a theory. I find this other approach less restraining and more multi-dimensional, one which draws on the whole image. When this image suddenly coalesces, the solution often comes in a flash of insight.

Coincidentally, I have always had an interest in food and metabolism. In fact, over the years, my M.D. brother, Robert Selby, and I had routinely traded and argued our own analyses and speculations about the latest research in the effect of nutrition on health and longevity. As a professor of medicine at the University of Arizona, Robert had access to extensive professional online databases which supplied a continuous source of new information he liked to pass on to me.

So as I drove home, pondering my dilemma, key pieces of data were beginning to take shape in my hologram. They were nebulous, but tantalizing. And coming in and out of focus at the center was the principle of metabolism, how our bodies change the food we eat into energy.

The inventor's hologram takes form

The clues that inspired a new solution

In thinking back to how my hologram came into focus, I realize that there were two critical pieces of anecdotal information which were floating in the foreground of my mind.

"Aha, we've been doing it wrong... what we need is a lot more —not less— fat."

The first was that when people lose weight, their LDL cholesterol levels drop helterskelter. Yet, when dieting stops at the desired weight the LDLs rise back to their pre-diet levels. For this reason, doctors who monitor weight-loss give limited importance to these readings. Instead of seeing this type of LDL drop as meaningless, I found it intriguing. The body is too magnificent a piece of engineering to label this erratic response as unreliable data. I sensed that there had to be a mechanism involved.

Another significant clue for me to consider was the fact that LDLs also come down with vigorous exercise. When exercising the body needs all the energy it can get. Metabolizing carbohydrates is not enough so it also needs to metabolize and mobilize fats.

What happens to the serum, or blood system, I wondered? Both when you lose weight and when you exercise you are dissolving the fat layer, or lipids, in your body. To create energy for the cells you need to get these lipids into the blood system to deliver them to the mitochondria, the body's "batteries". In other words, the lipids are being metabolized, that is, being broken down and transformed into energy. Hmm, cholesterol is a lipid...

I realized that the first and second observations about LDL drops had one thing in common: both weight loss and exercise cause the body to go into lipid, or fat, metabolism for energy. Instead of storing fat, the body burns it. So instead of storing cholesterol, would not lipid metabolism burn the cholesterol too?

Images and thoughts began to flow through my head... cholesterol... lipids... metabolism... lipid metabolism... how to activate it...*aha, we've been doing it wrong... what we need is a lot more— not less—fat.*

"Aha!" insight about fat

Burn fat—including cholesterol—with fat

On went the light bulb in my head. It lit up a vision of that metabolic pathways chart. I realized the solution to my problem was to activate the lipid metabolism.

And to do that we needed to keep up the lipid level in the body. In other words, replace carbohydrates with fats as the source of calories, and thereby energy, for the body.

A high-fat diet? This concept was sacrilege to the medical world, counter-intuitive to accepted theory. Fat is so often seen as the culprit in high cholesterol levels. "Low-fat" has been our modern mantra. But to a non-physician who looked at the science from a different angle, high fat made perfect sense. **It has not been scientifically proven that high fat in the diet is a culprit. It is only guilty by association: if high fat goes into the body we have just assumed it is converted to body fat.**

Instead, I theorized, the key to keeping the fat burners going is to increase, not decrease, the amount of fat in our diet. By making fat rather than carbohydrates the staple for providing calories for the body, we can ensure a continuous lipid metabolism. And, in so doing, we should get LDL reductions.

I decided what I needed to try was not just more fat, but a very high level of fats or lipids in my diet.

I theorized that this would push my body as far into the lipid metabolism mode as possible. In so doing, it would create the perfect environment for the consumption of lipoproteins in my blood, the complexes of lipid and protein which are the way lipids travel in the blood.

I believed that the interaction between lipids and lipoproteins would result, in simplified terms, in a sort of mill that would grind up and eat bad cholesterol, essentially the small-particle LDLs which are waste-products and get stuck in our arteries. I was already meditating and exercising, so I assumed that if I got the food aspect right, the body would repair itself. It could and would make the good cholesterol it needed.

The solution was inside my mind. Likewise, the power to heal my cholesterol imbalance on its own was inside my body.

Creating the formula

What to put in and what to keep out

With all those thoughts turning around in my head, I soon arrived home from the doctor's. I walked into the kitchen, reached for an apple, and announced to my wife, "You know, I think I should be able to change the metabolic pathways in my body. And I bet I can do it with food."

Before I could explain to her about the frightening calcium test results and my new mission, I was calling her over to the computer. "Linda! Come look at what the metabolic pathways chart looks like now!" It was a dense maze, packed with newly identified pathways, compared to the much simpler form I had last seen so many years ago. Now there were hundreds of different pathways added to the chart. But the key parts I was concerned about still matched what I had used back in college over forty years ago.

I studied the chart, felt satisfied with what I wanted to check, and decided not to do any additional research beyond what I already knew. I reached into the refrigerator to pull out some salad greens and squeezed some limes and poured olive oil on them.

Within two hours, I had my new diet designed and I had already put myself on it.

From that basic insight about the need for more than less fat—to keep fat burning—I started to quickly put together more of the pieces of my diet.

I remembered a couple of other clues from my inventor-style hologram of knowledge. One was the fact that high-glycemic foods, that is, foods which put high levels of sugar in the bloodstream rapidly, spike insulin levels in the body so that the burning of fat, or lipid metabolism, is shut down and storage of fat is induced. Most of the cells in our bodies can get their energy from either carbohydrates or fat. In America, it comes from plenty of foods which zoom into the bloodstream as one form of sugar or another. Pasta, potatoes, pizza, sodas, crackers, breakfast cereal, bread. Our body converts their starches and other carbohydrates into sugar. I knew that as long as the body is burning sugars, it will not do much to burn off fat. Instead, it stores fat in our fat cells... and it turns any carbohydrates that we have not burned yet into fat, i.e. lipids, as well.

Burning fat burns cholesterol. Eating sugar stops fat from burning. These were the headlines pulsating out of my hologram.

"Arthritis is obviously related to an inflammation in the body. Most people do not realize that obesity also is."

The other clue was something I remembered reading many years ago when my nieces and nephews were being given steroids for ear infections, a common medical problem in infants and toddlers. It seemed that ear infections were reduced by about 90% in one research study by removing fresh milk products and grains from the diet, because these products cause mild, chronic inflammation resulting in blockage of the small child's Eustachian tubes. Since heart disease is an inflammatory-related disease, I took anything that was pro-inflammatory out of the diet. I suspected that inflammation would raise levels of the "bad" cholesterol, the LDL.

My strategy then was to *make fats the primary source of calories, so the body would be forced to burn lipids, such as cholesterol, for energy.* I centered my new diet plan around olive oil, which I had learned to love on my bicycle trips to Italy. I decided that *"healthy" fats, in the form of oil or foods like nuts and avocados, would make up at least 65% of my calories.* I chose this number to be assured of robust lipid metabolism, yet still leaving enough room for a large amount and variety of vegetables and fruits. Olive oil and other fats would become the new staple of my diet, rather than the usual carbohydrates like bread, pasta or rice.

I next figured out how much protein I needed. I wanted just enough to maintain my muscles, bone and so on, but not more, since any extra protein just turns into sugar and nitrogen compounds. That meant *limiting protein to 15% of my total calories.* Egg whites and Greek-style strained yogurt as well as tofu were the main protein sources. (After a few days I found I could drop the protein to 10% and still do hard bicycle rides on a daily basis.)

So the balance would be made up of carbohydrates. Some intuitive sense and "grandmother wisdom" of "eat your spinach" and "an apple a day" were applied to my choice of carbohydrates. *All monocot grains, such as wheat, rice, and oats, as well as dairy were out because they were strong suspects in promoting inflammation*, as you will read later in this book. They were also eliminated because *I did not want high-glycemic foods*—meaning things that hit the bloodstream as sugar soon after they have been eaten. So out went not just grains and milk, but also potatoes, bananas, watermelon, and fruit juices. I would fill my plate instead with greens and raw fruit that are slow to release their sugars and are rich in fiber and beneficial phytochemicals, such as antioxidants to protect against cell damage. Salad greens, chard, kale, bok choy, broccoli, apples, blueberries and raspberries were examples of what would become my source of carbohydrates. *Carbs would make up only 20% of my new regimen, to keep me out of carbohydrate metabolism.*

Besides 65% lipids, 20% low Glycemic-index carbs and 15% protein, I limited my protocol to foods with no or very low cholesterol content and set fiber content to 35 grams or more to absorb any unused cholesterol (in the form of bile salts/sterols) in the gut that would be reabsorbed by the body.

A calorie-managed diet with high fat content, just enough protein to meet protein needs and the balance made up of non-grain, non-starchy carbohydrates. All in very specific proportions

Last, but not least, I decided to monitor the total amount of food I was eating. After all, if I wanted to burn off the extra LDLs in my blood, I figured it would happen faster if I did not eat too much. I set my target at 1200 calories because I wanted to lose a little weight at the same time. (For people trying our protocol, you will see that this level changes according to weight loss or gain goals.) I theorized that even if I could eat more calories and not gain weight, the body would just take the carbs for energy and not need the lipids. The whole point was to get the body to pick the lipids to burn.

So now I had it – ***a calorie-managed diet with high fat content, just enough***

protein to meet protein needs and the balance made up of non-grain, non-starchy carbohydrates. All in very specific proportions. My inventor's hologram had delivered a diet to reduce my cholesterol.

It had been two hours since I left the doctor's office. I was now ready to step into my new lab—my kitchen—and start becoming my own test subject.

"As an inventor with a background in biochemistry and technology, I found my dilemma frightening, yet at the same time fascinating."

CHAPTER 2

Worked the first time!

"Bad" LDLs -42, "good" HDLs +19 in 10 days

Myself as guinea pig

It was a simple, but not an easy, diet. I had created a specific formula using everyday food and was going to meticulously follow it so I could gauge how well it worked. The scientist's approach to collecting data, in other words.

That meant I carried a food scale around with me and carefully measured and weighed all my food down to the gram.

I also logged every bite I ate.

Then, from either labels or the Internet, I laboriously hand calculated the percentages of fats, protein, and carbohydrates in whatever amount of each food item I had put into my mouth.

My kitchen counters soon became cluttered and shirt pockets stuffed with scraps of paper covered in arithmetic. Several times a day I did a tally to see where my daily totals stood. At the end of the day, all numbers had to balance and fit into the formula I was testing for myself: 1200 total calories of which at least 65% of my calories coming from fats, about 10-15% from protein, 20% from carbohydrates.

After a couple days of sugar confusion in my body adjusting to turning to fats instead of carbs for energy, I found that my energy recovered and was even better than before. I was still beating people in my bicycling group. I was also enjoying foraging for new kinds of greens and found that dousing all my food with olive oil made it delicious (great carrier for spices) and very filling. This was not a deprivation diet and I felt great.

Still, I had trepidation about this dramatic metabolic shift. Would my fingers turn green or all my hair fall out?

I talked about the first phase of inventing, when you avoid looking into what is already known and accepted—as well as what is thought of as "impossible" or all the reasons why your proposed solution "won't work."

Now that I was more than half way into my experiment it was time to find out if anyone else had tried something similar and what kind of effects or results were produced.

So, on Day 6 of my diet, I headed off to the Boulder Bookstore and spent the whole day going through every single diet and health book I could find. I bought a dozen of them to bring home to read in detail. I had always thought of most diet books as fads without much scientific substance, but as I read through them, I found myself impressed by pearls of wisdom scattered here and there, sometimes where I least expected.

I did not find any books, however, which set out to reduce cholesterol the way I was doing. They were primarily geared toward weight loss, and any dealing with cholesterol reduction produced the slow rate associated with simply losing weight. That meant long-term programs with relatively modest improvements.

> *"Everyone has a doctor in him or her; we just have to help it in its work. The natural healing force within each one of us is the greatest forces in getting well."*
>
> - Hippocrates

Most importantly, there was nothing that caused me to change my course. I continued reaching for walnuts and avocados instead of muffins and loading my plate with salad greens and vegetables grilled in olive oil instead of pasta in creamy Alfredo sauce. And I kept measuring, logging and calculating throughout the day.

Moment of truth

LDLs down 42 and HDLs up 19 points in 10 days

My doctor had given me two weeks to prove that I did not need a prescription for statins. So after ten days on the diet, I called the clinic and left word that I wanted a blood test for cholesterol. A different doctor,

Let's add dark chocolate

whom I did not know, called me back.

"You just had a test two weeks ago, and you want another one?" asked this other doctor.

"Yes," I said. "I've developed a new diet, and I'm hoping some things have changed for the better."

"You guys change your diet and you do a little exercise and you think everything is going to be OK, and that's just not the case," the doctor sighed. "This stuff changes very slowly and it's way too soon for any improvements to show up."

The doctor said he would not approve another blood test for at least another six months.

So maybe I was naïve, but I still was curious to see if any change had happened in this short time.

"OK, thank you," I said, just before heading to a lab where I could get the blood test on my own as long as I paid for it myself.

The next morning, I picked up the test results and set off for the Trident Café to join my morning coffee group. I sat down, espresso in hand, and looked at my numbers. I could not believe what I was seeing.

My LDLs had gone down from 117 to 75 and my HDLs had gone up from 84 to 103. In ten days.

I had been simply hoping my two-week experiment would produce some kind of change showing a trend for the better. What I got instead was an astonishing 42 mg/dl drop in my LDLs and 19mg/dl increase in my HDLs.

You might recall my earlier reference to the recent *New England Journal of Medicine* study comparing the three most popular diets of today: the American Heart Association low-fat diet, the Mediterranean, and the Atkins low-carb. The best they did in reducing LDL cholesterol was a decrease of 4.3 mg/dl in six months.

I was surprised by how fast my diet had worked—and how unbelievably well. This was my only invention that worked the first time around!

Victory whoop in the coffee shop

Success attracts recruits

I let out a "WOW!!!" and everyone within earshot wanted to know why I was so excited. For the next half hour I had a dozen people sitting around me listening to how I had dramatically changed my cholesterol numbers in less than two weeks. Every one of them either had some cholesterol problem, or had someone in the family with a problem, and several of them were on cholesterol-lowering drugs. Cholesterol had not even been on my radar before the heart calcium scan which had set off this chain of events. I was surprised to see how many people worried about cholesterol and statins.

I immediately called my M.D. brother Robert to ask him about my amazing results. He jumped into a role of becoming my biggest skeptic, my toughest peer reviewer, and, at other times, advisor and cheerleader. I told him I was going to see if I could duplicate my results, and he suggested adding dark chocolate for its role in increasing HDL "good" cholesterol. That, of course, was not a difficult decision, so I included chocolate (or more precisely, non-alkalized cocoa) in my new dietary protocol.

My friend Mel, a physicist and fellow private pilot, was due for his flight physical, and he wanted to improve his cholesterol profile. His HDLs were low. In addition, his doctor wanted him to get his LDLs below 100 mg/dl and he had never been able to do so, even though he had always been a serious exercise fanatic all his life. He asked if I could help him, and I said I would be happy to show him what I had done.

Then my wife, who has been slim all her life and who liked to eat leftover chocolate mousse for breakfast, happened to get her physical and was shocked to find that she now had high cholesterol.

Within two weeks of going on my diet, both of my new experimentees saw the same kind of results I did, despite not being as consistent as I was for the whole period (wives and friends do not tend to automatically comply with what you request). Mel's HDLs went up 14 mg/dl and he got his LDL level down to 89, just like he wanted, while my wife reduced her LDLs by an impressive 50 mg/dl.

Soon, after seeing these results, other members of our "Trident Gang" were clamoring to be guinea pigs too.

CHAPTER 3

High fives beyond cholesterol

Discovery of bonus health benefits of the BalancePoint diet and making them available to everyone

3000 articles and a 118-year-old man later

Studying the literature and setting up scientific models

Before I started signing up more would-be dieters, I told them to let me do a little more research and get a few more support tools in place. I wanted to see if anyone was doing this kind of high-lipid research and I also wanted to know more about results from other types of similar studies. I headed off to the University of Colorado library where I had spent countless nights in the biochemistry stacks decades ago.

Once again I found myself ensconced in the library until closing time each evening. I did this for six weeks. This time around, though, the medical articles were available online, giving me unimaginable access to up-to-the-minute research from around the world. During this time I scanned about 3000 medical and scientific journal abstracts and read about 250 articles.

I did not find anything with data coming close to our remarkable results. What I did find was confirmation of my hunches but in bits and pieces. There were hints throughout the literature, but no one had put all the parts of the puzzle together into one approach for rapidly reducing cholesterol like my diet.

It seemed like heresy at this time to suggest that high fat content would be beneficial for people, yet I could see fingers pointing this way throughout history.

One major study that jumped out at me was the ground-breaking "Seven Country Study" by Ancel Keys, who looked at the correlation between what we eat and how we fare heart health-wise in contrasting populations around the world between 1958 and 1970. Finland had the highest incidence of cardiovascular events: 152 for every 33 events of the Mediterranean countries.

On the Greek island of Crete, however, the number was only three. Heart problems were almost unheard of. This was a fact I later confirmed for myself *fig. 4*

AVERAGE REDUCTIONS AFTER 2 WEEKS ON BALANCEPOINT

Total cholesterol ↓56 mg/dl
LDL cholesterol ↓52 mg/dl
Triglycerides ↓30 mg/dl
Arterial age equivalency ↓19 years
Weight ↓8 lb*

**For those wanting to lose weight—not necessary for above reductions*
Source: "Dietary Protocol for a Rapid Reduction of Risk Levels of Cholesterols, Triglycerides and Arterial Stiffness: a Before/After Study of a Pilot Dietary Program." For full table of results see Appendix 1 of this book.

when this first phase of my BalancePoint research prompted me to take my family on a trip to Crete. We met people like the lady selling shoes to my teenage daughter who told us we just missed meeting her grandfather. He had recently died at age 118, but his sister was still very much alive at 105! Keys noted how the Cretans "put olive oil on everything," including their breakfast, and he was puzzled that they still did not have heart disease.

Another pointer toward the benefit of high fats appeared while I was giving my Trident gang updates on my literature search. One of the group members brought me a worn-out diet book he had scavenged from a tenant's throw-away pile. I was going to jettison the book too as soon as my friend left. But then, as I politely flipped through the book, I came across the interesting research of a scientist named Vilhjalmur Stefansson. He studied another group of people who were traditionally strangers to heart disease, the Canadian Inuit along the Arctic Ocean. They centered their diet on whale and seal blubber. I remembered on reading this that when I had once gone on a dogsled and igloo trip with the Inuit, I found it curious that they gave most of the caribou meat to their dogs and would keep fatty organs, like the liver, to eat themselves.

This led me on a trail of articles about our ancestral hunter-gatherers, who similarly ate mostly the fat-laden organs of wild animals, and also did not suffer from heart disease and strokes.

These findings, as well as others described later in Part III, provided evidence that a high-fat diet had been successfully used among different populations and cultures. I gained enough comfort to let my friends try it too.

I wanted to monitor participants from a medical standpoint, so I recruited my friend Dr. John O'Hearne, an M.D. in Internal Medicine in Boulder, to scrutinize their data. John was focusing on preventative medicine and had heart patient management experience with Dr. Dean Ornish's pioneering lifestyle program for reversing heart disease. Though the Ornish program is famous as a low-fat diet, John saw very quickly from our results how a diet on the opposite spectrum, one with a high fat content, could have a great deal of power for reversing the risk of heart disease.

I next arranged to send my dieters to the Boulder Community Hospital Laboratory to measure their blood chemistry before and after going on the two-week diet.

I assigned each participant a total daily intake of calories. Soon, the members of my first group of cholesterol-busters were scrupulously measuring everything they ate on their digital food scales, according to my very exact rules for type of food and quantity. They even carried with them a little pre-measured container of olive oil to make sure they were getting the required amount every day.

High fives for everyone

Consistent 30-40 point drops in LDLs

After finishing the two-week program, each participant eagerly went into the lab for blood tests. The results were profound.

You could hear the cheers and see us high-fiving each other as each new set of results came in. **Everyone who stuck to the diet saw unheard-of improvements in their cholesterol numbers—a 40 to 50 mg/dl drop in bad LDL cholesterol in two weeks. Even those who were on cholesterol-reducing statin drugs saw the same reductions.** It was obvious, then, that the diet offered a different mechanism than statins so the effect was additive.

One participant who had battled cholesterol problems for decades, and was unable to take cholesterol-lowering drugs, dropped her LDL cholesterol number by 81 mg/dl—going from 151 to 70.

However, it was not just the LDLs that were being affected.

Triglycerides, another type of lipid whose excessively high levels can be associated with heart disease risk, were also reduced. Again, with significant reductions. One person dropped her triglycerides by 84 mg/dl in just four days.

And the level of good cholesterol, HDLs, increased for some people, especially when the numbers were low to begin with.

Incidentally, statin drugs suppress the production of LDLs and so reduce

When my doctor in Alabama saw my blood test results after going on BalancePoint, she said, "I put a lot of people on all kinds of diets, and, sure, they end up losing weight. But this is a diet where you actually get healthy!"

Mike S., Age 66

their levels, but generally do not affect triglycerides or HDLs.

It was becoming clear that the **cholesterol was not just being reduced—it was being put back into balance.**

I overheard my doctor brother Robert, after seeing these results, give this perspective of my discovery: *"Along comes this crazy inventor who doesn't know any better so he designs a high-fat diet."*

Our test results were exciting enough that Robert flew in to hear me present my results to Dr. Robert Eckel, who was at that time President of the American Heart Association and on faculty at the University of Colorado School of Medicine. We talked about the massive "Nurses Study" which had recently documented that a low-fat diet did not reduce the heart attack risk of the study's participants. I suggested that they turn the question upside down—and look at the "cheaters" who ate a high fat diet. As it turns out, an analysis later did come out in a study which showed that those who did eat more fat actually showed lower incidence of heart disease.

Anti-inflammatory benefits start appearing

Weight loss, decrease in arthritic pain, reversal of inflammation of the arteries

As more people tried our program, they were reporting even more surprises—the ones who wanted to lose weight were accomplishing it, even on a high-fat diet. They were losing about five to ten pounds in the first two weeks alone. And they were losing belly fat, which is the most dangerous type of fat and the most difficult to lose.

It is important to point out that those people who did not want to lose weight did not have to, and they still got the same cholesterol reduction results. This outcome contradicted the common doctor's refrain that we were getting LDL decreases simply through weight loss. (Besides, the LDL reductions you get from weight loss do not begin to approach the magnitude and speed of the reduction seen on the BalancePoint diet.) We were finding that people were able to manage their weight profile as they wished, to either maintain, gain or lose weight, and still get the same cholesterol benefits.

Also, our early participants noted that long-time problems with allergies or arthritis were much better. One woman noted that she was not doing her yoga in the morning any more, and I wondered how our diet kept her from this routine. Then she explained that she no longer had the arthritic pain that prompted her to do yoga exercises each day. I then realized that I too was not experiencing aches in my ankles from a big fall, and had just done a long hike without discomfort.

Anecdotal reports like this led me back to an earlier train of thought—I had selected some foods and banished others in order to reduce the chance of inflammation caused by the foods people ate. That was a big reason for leaving out grains and dairy, for instance.

Arthritis is obviously related to an inflammation in the body. Most people do not realize that obesity also is. (You will see in Part III how medical researchers are beginning to attribute most age-related chronic illnesses to an inflammatory response in the body.)

A new question popped into my mind: Inflammation has been correlated to heart disease and potential for strokes. Could the diet be helping, in some direct way, to actually reverse this disease (called ASCVD, arteriosclerotic cardiovascular disease)?

I looked for a way to measure the diet's direct effect on these risks. And I wanted a non-invasive way—the diet participants were not about to volunteer for more needle pricks for blood tests, with one of my more game experimentees already calling himself "Binx's pincushion."

Another doctor friend of mine provided the answer. He happened to connect me with nationally recognized imaging expert, Dr. James Ehrlich, M.D., of Colorado Heart Imaging and faculty member of medical schools at the University of Colorado School and George Washington University.

Using Dr. Ehrlich's medical testing instrument called a Sphygmocor, we started doing readings of aortic augmentation pressure and augmentation index to measure the stiffness of the arteries and vascular system. The importance of stiffness can be understood by thinking about "hardening of the arteries." Many health professionals believe that as we get older, our blood vessels are doomed to harden, thus becoming easier to damage. Stiffer blood vessels can also lead to higher blood pressure.

{ *Not all LDLs are bad.* }

Why is this stiffness a measure of inflammation in the arteries—and probably other parts of the body as well? Envision how a rash develops when your skin gets inflamed, and the skin gets thicker and less elastic. It is a similar process in the arteries.

Arteries 30 years younger

When we tested the blood vessels of our diet participants, the results were just as startling and rewarding as we had found with cholesterol testing.

People on our diet were showing the cardiovascular health age equivalence of people 10-30 years younger than their chronological age. Their arteries were getting younger in age.

Dr. Ehrlich was so impressed that he also tried the BalancePoint diet because, when he was demonstrating his arterial stiffness-measuring instrument to us, it showed him with a cardiovascular age equivalency of a 75-year-old. He was 54 at the time. Having the technology at hand in his office, he could not resist testing himself after only three days on the diet. He found in that short time the stiffness of his blood vessels had already begun to reverse, and they now had the flexibility of a 43-year-old.

"Aha" about the cause of inflammation

It was this extraordinarily rapid response produced by only a few days on our diet that made me realize there is only one thing which could change so quickly—inflammation.

It began the investigation and confirmation of my suspicions that **our**

diet's true power was in its anti-inflammatory nature.

It is known that inflammation causes heart disease. It was assumed that cholesterol triggered the inflammation. Our observations pointed me in the opposite direction.

This study brought me to an "Aha!" more significant than the one about keeping the body in lipid metabolism. I realized that a previously unheard-of cholesterol-inflammation sequence is involved. It is what we eat which activates the chronic inflammation related to cardiovascular disease. This food-induced chronic inflammation opens the walls of the arteries to allow infiltration of small particle-size LDL cholesterol to initiate the problems leading to heart attacks and stroke. (The chronic inflammation also promotes the development of a whole series of diseases.) Chapters 8 and 9 explain in more detail how I came into this insight.

And, as you read on, you will find even more intriguing and significant results along the way.

Targeting the real villains

Decrease of small-particle LDLs

We soon discovered that not only can our diet lower cholesterol at least as well as a statin drug, it targets the specific type of LDL which is the problematic contributor to heart disease.

It turns out that not all LDLs are "bad" (I actually do not like the terms "bad" or "good" because everything in the body has a function

COMPARISON TO OTHER DIETS

Remember what I said earlier about our minds wanting to fit things into comfortable categories and 'boxes"? It is not surprising that people continually want to describe or compare BalancePoint in relation to other well-known diets. So let's do a quick review.

Many would like to pigeonhole BalancePoint as a modified Mediterranean diet. However, we use twice the amount of fat (65-70%) and we do not use grains—two significant differences. Others might compare us to low-carb diets. Again, we differ in our very high fat content. Also, low-carb diets tend to advocate large amounts of protein and often no fruit, both of which are not the case with BalancePoint.

The most important difference between BalancePoint and any diet, though, comes down to two issues:

1. BalancePoint is a specific formula. We find that there is a small envelope of tolerance around this formula to get the spectacular type of results we

are known for. Any deviations from this formula may give results other diets would be thrilled with, such as a 20 mg/dl reduction in LDLs, but not the incredible 40-70 mg/dl LDL decreases we see in two weeks. There are layers of science built into our need for precision in this protocol. That is how we get the expected outcomes.

2 After two weeks, we find that BalancePoint participants show not just one but many risk factors in cardiovascular and metabolic areas not simply improving, but achieving optimum healthy status. In Figure 4, you can see that LDLs, triglycerides, blood pressure, and glucose are now in the optimal range after only two weeks. For some people, it's the first time in decades. We have not seen any other diet match these results.

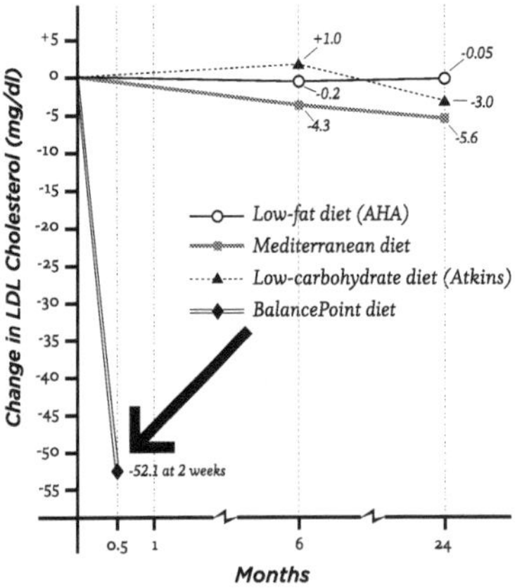

fig. 1.2

and we just are not smart enough to know all we need to know about all these parts.) Anyway, the "large, fluffy" LDLs are actually needed by the body for muscle and other cellular repair. It is their waste products, the so-called "small particle" LDLs which are small enough to penetrate the artery walls and damage the arteries.

When we started sending in blood samples of our diet participants to a lab for sophisticated NMR (Nuclear Magnetic Resonance) analysis showing particle sizes, the reports indicate that our diet lowers the number of small particle LDLs and leaves the large, fluffy ones alone. Statins work by interrupting the natural pathway of making LDLs, and so suppresses both the beneficial large fluffy ones and the small particle ones.

In other words, this dietary protocol has a better overall result than cholesterol drugs.

What's in a name?

With all the interest in my diet, I started exploring how to help people do the protocol well. After hearing a diet participant ask another if she was, 'Binxing' it today? I knew I needed a name other than the "Binx" diet. I chose the name BalancePoint.

For me, "BalancePoint" comes from the stability of a triangle, a figure with three important elements: diet, stress management, and exercise. All three are necessary components for the kind of lifestyle change which leads to better health, a lifestyle which produces the environment for the body to repair itself.

Our focus right now, of course, is diet.

Since 2006, we have tested a few hundred diet participants and each of these has undoubtedly shared the protocol with other family members and friends. We found that we could reproduce the same LDL reductions for everyone who complied with my strict two-week dietary formula: an average of 40-50 mg/dl decrease for about 85% of those compliant with the protocol.

People have been achieving not only desired health goals in the two weeks. They are also noticing a newfound sense of intuitive eating—of letting their body tell them which foods are good for them and how much or little they need. They are set for launching the BalancePoint Wellness Lifestyle which will maintain their new results.

Which foods to keep in or out of the diet?

The diet has barely changed from the original one I devised in my Eureka moment when faced with the prospect of taking drugs for the rest of my life. We keep fine-tuning the protocol, but the changes have been very minor. For instance, I added the cocoa for its flavanols to raise HDLs, and I included wine for its resveratrol component, which is being studied for cardiovascular benefits.

It does not hurt that people like to say, "A diet which includes chocolate and wine is my kind of diet!"

Grains, sad to say, are one of the prime culprits.

Then when we experimented with removing or adding foods to this formula with our first group of people, we found that any grains, whether "healthy" steel-cut oatmeal and coarse-grain breads or Italian risotto, raised LDLs back to close to previous levels and dramatically increased arterial stiffness in just days. Meat, however, had a lesser negative effect.

After finding this negative effect of grains on cholesterol of our protocol participants, I started to come across interesting work on the problem with grains. I found literature by someone who happened to live in my back yard, a scientist named Loren Cordain from Fort Collins, Colorado. Around the same time, I was reading a *Science* journal article about work done by Swedish medical researchers on a protein called a "lectin" in grains. As you will see in Part III about why BalancePoint works, the research done on lectins gives interesting theories of why grains can cause inflammation.

People always ask if they need to keep to the same food list after the two-week program. The answer is basically, "yes." However, the protein can come from different sources, such as grass-fed animals, as long as the proportions of fat/protein/carbs remains the same and the portions remain low. There are also other allowances as described in Part IV, The BalancePoint Protocol. You will be able to tell yourself how you are being affected by the introduction of a new food.

But this is where we could do a lot of research.

There are so many questions I want to explore. I'd like to correlate, for example the effect of more types of foods on the cardiometabolic biomarkers, such as cholesterol levels, arterial stiffness, blood pressure, glucose readings, and weight. Also, one of the key questions about any diet is its sustainability. We have people who have successfully maintained their weight and lipid profiles after several years: how rigorously do they maintain their lifestyle change?

A most exciting research area is the use of protein arrays to characterize gene expression. Our research suggests that in most cases our protocol produces results even if you have a genetic propensity for a particular disease, like high cholesterol.

Collaboration with doctors and researchers

My interest as a scientist has always been in research. This led me to form a non-profit institute, the Lifestyle for Health Research Institute, to promote research into nutritional and lifestyle solutions to atherosclerotic cardiovascular disease and metabolic syndrome. The institute is a coalition of medical and scientific researchers and physicians interested in non-drug solutions which are affordable and sustainable for healthy aging and the prevention and treatment of metabolic, cardiovascular and inflammatory-related health problems.

The current focus is to research how the BalancePoint diet can prevent and help solve conditions such as cholesterol imbalance and metabolic syndrome, which is a set of risk factors including abdominal obesity, elevated blood pressure, insulin resistance or glucose intolerance, low HDLs and high triglycerides in cholesterol. (Metabolic syndrome is an increasingly common condition which afflicts more than 50 million Americans and puts them at risk of heart disease, diabetes, and a host of other illnesses. The incidence of Type 2 Diabetes, for example, has doubled in the U.S. in just ten years.) Our results have been of great interest to the medical doctors and researchers we showed them to, and soon, my personal physician was sending us clients. So too has the doctor who had told me once, "It takes years to lower cholesterol!" Cardiologists are now working with us to implement programs using the BalancePoint protocol as a preventative approach to cardiovascular disease. We have given presentations of our research to the heads of top medical schools in the country, such as the University of Chicago, as well as to professional associations like the American College of Cardiology.

I have talked about how, over the years, there have been many hints that a high-lipid diet showed promise. Despite this, no one had pursued it clinically. Some studies had looked at parts of the approach, but **I found none that put it all together. And nothing suggested anything near the early results we had**.

The best solutions are those which in hindsight seem so simple and so obvious. Now that the BalancePoint formula is successful, people can point to scientific papers that support elements of our protocol.

When I described the invention of the diet earlier, I talked about the difference in thinking approaches between the usual compulsion to simplify, categorize and explain versus a more intuitive, holistic approach. People know that the diet worked the first time, and has continued to work in the same basic format for almost everyone since then. The question often comes up, "But why does it work?" We all want to put things into the frameworks we understand.

Wellness means living well

I am intrigued by the mechanism of the diet, and that is the focus of my theoretical research interest. I am finding new clues to help fill in the blanks.

It is interesting that in the last few years, new research has emerged to offer more pieces of the puzzle, each with their different takes on the problem. Most of this research offers theories and speculation. We are delighted that we can offer actual data—data of how some of these theories have actually proven themselves "in the field," so to speak, with our diet participants. Medical researchers have been excited to find out about our data and results, and we are working on collaborating with them so we can all work together in leading edge research. Our ongoing, extensive database detailing the food input down to the gram level and its correlation to various biomarkers is of great interest to these researchers.

Our goal with this book

I can say that after over six years of eating BalancePoint-style, my cholesterol levels are still great, I still bicycle in the foothills, and my ankles ache only on the few occasions when I cannot resist that bite of bran muffin. As for the scary calcium score that started this adventure, I took a second test and there was no additional accumulation of calcium in my arteries, so those first deposits may have happened even decades ago. But it served its purpose in launching this diet and book, which I hope will help many.

This is the story of how BalancePoint evolved from a hunch by a panicked inventor who was desperate to lower his cholesterol into a nutritional lifestyle embraced not only by medical professionals but also top chefs who have taken my rudimentary diet to gastronomic heights. Cavemen who thrived on roots and berries probably never imagined dried cherry duck breast with cold mint salad.

Like some of my friends who see me chortling over our newest blood test results at the local coffee shop and want to know the details, you can delve into my scientific discourse, which I will describe in the chapters that follow.

Or you can grasp the basics, skip to the recipe section and head for your kitchen.

At the very least, we hope to inspire you with our basic premise: "Wellness means living well." At the most, we want you to join with us in the journey to discovering how well our bodies are meant to work, when we learn to treat them right.

The common response of people trying BalancePoint is their joy in discovering that they are in control. They can control aspects of their health they never thought possible before—cardiovascular health, weight, metabolic health. As one man said, "I feel I'm in the driver's seat now."

It is as simple as that, and what worthier result than taking back control of your health and living?

"Burning fat burns cholesterol. Eating sugar stops fat from burning."

PART THREE

Reversing inflammation—the science behind BalancePoint

Our breakthrough discovery and why BalancePoint works!

The "orchestra" playing in our body called the human genome and what we need to do to tune it... the rapid cholesterol results confirming success in resetting metabolic pathways to perform better... reduction of stiffness in the arteries to make them 20 years-younger in just days... the use of fats to keep our body burning fat and cholesterol... the problem with newcomers to the human diet, such as foods which do not make the body work hard enough to digest them and grains with their built in "poison pill protein"... the reason why the conventional approach of just lowering cholesterol numbers is not a solution... BalancePoint's new insight to explain how food-induced mild, chronic inflammation causes heart and metabolic disease... these are all pieces that contribute to the layers that make up the BalancePoint protocol.

Our data is our science layer. We have clinically proven results unlike anything that has ever been seen regarding the speed and

FLY THE PLANE "INSIDE THE ENVELOPE"

The story of the science behind the BalancePoint diet starts with the human genome—our complete set of DNA.

Left to itself, the human genome is a rather elegant blueprint and operator's manual for how the body should work. It represents a balance point wherein the body can maintain a state of wellness.

Pilots are familiar with the concept of operating an aircraft within its "envelope"—the set of technological limitations in which the aircraft can function safely and effectively. Keeping within recommended power settings and weight and balance

magnitude of cardiometabolic benefit from our protocol. We also have a precise formula and protocol plus a record of all food eaten—down to the gram level—by our participants in our 2-week Jumpstart program

BalancePoint returns biomarkers to normal within two weeks

What is even more significant than the amount of the LDL drops is that, in just two weeks, the biomarkers of the BalancePoint protocol participants in our study (*fig. 4*) came out with levels considered normal or healthy.

Regardless of what the actual change was, the biomarkers after our two-week program showed optimal levels for measurements such as non-HDL cholesterol (now considered a more accurate indicator of risk than LDL), triglycerides, stiffness of the arteries, and stabilizing of blood sugar levels.

It made no difference if the participants had a genetic predisposition to high cholesterol or if they were an elite athlete performing at an Olympic level. They were still able to come out of the two weeks with healthy numbers. These results also occurred in even those people who showed high-risk factors for heart disease or stroke when they came to BalancePoint.

We have continued to observe this pattern with the hundreds of people who have done the two-week protocol over the last three years.

This data was produced under carefully controlled conditions. Consequently, we have one other scientific contribution that

calculations are examples of taking care not to fly "outside the envelope." Otherwise, the aircraft's performance would be unpredictable and unreliable and can result in damage to the aircraft.

The same principle of functioning outside the envelope applies to our bodies. There are many things that we do as humans that can unbalance our biological systems, to force the body to function in ways for which it was not designed. Such malfunctioning can lead to abnormalities like cancer, heart disease, and diabetes.

But the important thing to remember is that the superbly designed blueprint or manual called the human genome is always there, ready to be activated. ***If we can produce the environment in which the genome can perform best, the body can fix itself. It can re-balance.***

BalancePoint creates that optimal environment. The body can set itself to work, and we each find our own unique balance point.

- Linda Jade Fong 2007

our research colleagues appreciate: a carefully recorded database noting the exact food intake, precise to the gram, of our participants and the correlating before and after medical test results.

One other important component of the science behind BalancePoint centers on our discovery of how to reset the metabolic pathways to keep the body burning fats instead of carbohydrates. In this way, the body keeps "eating" excess cholesterol and eliminates blood sugar spikes and valleys.

And the foundation for all of this is the powerful anti-inflammatory action of the BalancePoint diet. Our radical approach strikes at the root of many inflammatory-related problems, ranging from high cholesterol, obesity and heart disease to diabetes, allergies, arthritis—and also acne!

The next few chapters will focus on how our diet acts on the body's natural biochemistry to produce the results which made you pick up this book. The goal of this discussion is to provide you with:

- Science-based understanding of why we ask you to comply with some non-conventional aspects of the protocol, such as high fat and no grains, and their part in the relationship between inflammation and heart disease.
- Background for you and your doctor to understand how the BalancePoint diet fits in with, and provides a solution for, the newest medical research information and directives, such as the *2008 Consensus Statement from the American Diabetes Association and the American College of Cardiology Foundation*.
- Explanation of why our clinical experience with BalancePoint delivers such dramatic results and how it gives new insights into the causes of cardiovascular and metabolic disease as well as the role of the BalancePoint diet in preventing and healing these conditions

On average, people at the end of BalancePoint's two-week program show arteries like someone 20 years younger.

See Appendix 1

CHAPTER 4

Creating the environment in which the body can heal itself

Getting back to the "BalancePoint" designed by our genes

We have 20 to 25 thousand genes that make up our genome. They are like members of an orchestra. It is an orchestra so enormous that it holds all the genetic information and instructions for every type of cell in our body. (Yet at the same time it is miniature enough that the whole orchestra is tucked into each cell of our body.) Like every orchestra, this genome ensemble has a repertoire of classical music pieces that it knows how to play well. Now imagine suddenly demanding that these 20,000 to 25,000 classically-trained musicians improvise a piece of avant-garde jazz music or perform an ancient Balinese song using only traditional gamelan xylophones, drums and gongs. Different skills and knowledge are called for. The orchestra might be able to sort of play the new music, but it would not do it very well.

The reason we use the name BalancePoint for the diet is because it is about finding the lifestyle "sweet spot" in the genome [our personal genetic makeup]. It is the point where nutrition and the foods in our diet, plus activity and stress management, are optimized so that the genome can maintain optimal health.

This is what it is like when we take the genes that we have, which were developed over 50 million years of primate evolution, and ask them to operate on a completely different diet. (We will get into more details about this unfamiliar diet later.) Instead of the skills and capabilities that our body is used to performing with, it is being asked to abruptly improvise, to deal with being fed something it is not used to. We can expect it to function only marginally now, and this is why we end up having so many health problems and aging-related diseases.

When we are asking our genes to do something on a continual basis that they do not have the knowledge to deal with perfectly, we end up with imperfect operation: metabolism that is out of balance, repair that is inadequate, maintenance that is unsatisfactory, gene expression that is defective... The body knows how to perform all of these functions faultlessly—if provided with the music it knows how to play. In other words, if we have it do the repertoire it already knows. That is not to say that eventually it cannot replace its musicians, bring in new instruments, practice and learn new styles or music, but it takes thousands, even tens of thousands, of years. That is what happens—the genome eventually adapts, but over an evolutionary time span rather than in a few generations.

ALREADY ON STATINS?

People on statins can still go on the BalancePoint diet and benefit from it. They will get as rapid and significant a drop in their LDL numbers. Our diet participants on statins have consequently been able, under their doctor's supervision, to either decrease their dosage of statins or in some cases to completely go off them.

Because the effect of BalancePoint is additive, it is additional proof to us that a different mechanism is involved than that of statins.

We can keep eating the way we do and suffer the disease that results. Or we can change our lifestyle to accommodate the way the genome is designed and live longer, healthier lives. The BalancePoint philosophy is to help people get back to what our genes know how to do, what they know how to do best. Our genes can do this if we provide the foods, the physical activity levels, and the stress management that most closely conform to how our evolutionary history has designed us to operate. Then we can expect our bodies to perform well.

Let the body fix itself naturally

That is, in fact, how BalancePoint tackles our health problems, such as high cholesterol—by providing the environment for optimal body performance. By doing so, we allow the body to play its familiar repertoire which includes natural self-healing. It is really a very different approach than trying to understand and fix an individual element of the body's metabolism. That is how drugs are designed.

When our automatic response is to pull out a prescription pad whenever illness strikes us, I think there is something we have to keep in mind. The highly targeted approach of most medications is very difficult and rather tricky because the interrelationships of a body's orchestra are very complex. There are a multitude of feedback systems, interactions between genes, and interactions with environment and food type.

All of the above, working at different levels all at the same time, contribute to the intricacy of the operation of our bodies. It is very challenging to treat one thing, whether a specific biochemical pathway or symptom, and expect to solve the problem without affecting—or being affected by—other interactions. Finding the one drug to fix a particular symptom often produces mixed results or unintended consequences.

What we really need to do is switch our lifestyle to one that more closely matches the lifestyle under which we human beings evolved. This solution can have its limitations too—we cannot really make all of those changes becoming true hunter-gatherers out in the woods again. The good news is that we do not have to.

What we really need to do is switch our lifestyle to one that more closely matches the lifestyle under which we human beings evolved

There are three changes that seem to do the trick. An obvious one is that we need to make sure we have adequate physical activity in our lives.

Another is that we support our emotional well-being through stress management and strong family, community, or spiritual nurturing. (It is interesting to consider, for example, how much the very real benefits of the cultural tradition of eating together as a social activity have contributed to the historically positive effect of diets like the Mediterranean diet.)

The third requirement is to get our food intake to align more closely to the diet which has nurtured our development as

The end result of BalancePoint's nutritional shift is not only dramatically improved numbers on the lipid panel—such as cholesterol, triglycerides, amount of small particle LDLs—at the doctor's office. By addressing the root of the problem, chronic inflammation, BalancePoint is producing better numbers for people on a whole series of cardiometabolic biomarkers, including abdominal obesity; elevated blood pressure, insulin resistance or glucose intolerance.

a species. That, of course, is the focus of this book. BalancePoint will show you how simple but precise changes in your diet can bring about re-balancing in days.

So what happens when we try to operate "outside the envelope" we were designed for? Our systems get out of balance, and we begin to develop diseases which claim our lives or reduce our quality of life, such as cardiovascular disease, arthritis, and diabetes. These conditions are often associated with aging, and their onset may be very slow or, in some cases, very sudden.

The onset begins earlier than most of us realize. A 2008 study of young children showed that obese children as young as 10 had arteries as stiff as those of 45-year-olds.

Our results show that we can usually stop and probably even reverse this process in adults, and it would probably work in children as well.

CHAPTER 5

When "bad" does not necessarily mean "bad"

Almost everyone has a family member or close friend with a cholesterol problem. An important focus of the BalancePoint protocol and this book is, "Rapid Cholesterol Reduction," and most people are geared toward the notion of cholesterol as a villain. However, cholesterol itself is not the problem. Cholesterol is an essential building block of cell structure, including nerve cells, and of hormones. It is also vital for body repair and maintenance, and the digestion and absorption of fats. When cholesterol levels are too low people get symptoms like sore muscles and memory loss or forgetfulness.

To get to the many places in the body where it is needed, cholesterol must travel through the blood system. But cholesterol is a fat or, in medical terms, a lipid, so it is not soluble in aqueous solutions like blood. In order to be carried through our vascular system, it is surrounded by a protein (called ApoB). I like to describe this protein as the six-pack for carrying cholesterol through our bodies. The resulting macro-molecule made up of the carrier protein and its load of cholesterol is called a lipoprotein. The carrier protein has docking receptors which allow the lipoprotein to deliver its cargo to the sites where cholesterol is needed.

Technically speaking, the cholesterol test results you get from your doctor are really measurements of the whole lipoprotein, and not just the cholesterol payload. But since it is the cholesterol that doctors have focused on, everyone tends to refer to the lipoprotein as "cholesterol."

Your blood test results will show a measurement of total cholesterol, but this number is actually not very meaningful because it is the combined total of both the desired and less desired cholesterol components. That is why you will see your doctor study its breakdown into LDL and HDL cholesterol. LDL stands for "low density lipoprotein", generally dubbed as the so-called "bad" or less desired cholesterol, and HDL means "high density lipoprotein," known as the "good" cholesterol.

The unit of measurement is the number of milligrams (mg) per deciliter (dL) of blood. We all know that lowering the level of so-called "bad" cholesterol, and raising the level of "good" cholesterol will reduce our risk of heart disease. When your doctor tells you to get your LDLs below a certain point, such as 100 mg/dL, and HDLs above a specific number, such as >39 mg/dL, she is probably referring to a range that medical boards, such as the National Institutes of Health, have defined as a risk factor for cardiovascular disease.

The key to the BalancePoint approach is to re-balance the biochemistry in our body so that our metabolism can work at its best, in the way our genome or body "blueprint" wants it to.

I find that, in many ways, the labels "bad cholesterol" or "good cholesterol" are misleading. Our bodies—primarily the liver—manufacture LDLs for a very specific function Every cell in our body needs cholesterol for repair, maintenance and growth—and LDLs are the vehicles that transport the cholesterol. So that is an essential function. As soon as you interfere with that pathway, you are interfering with something that operates naturally to fulfill that important role.

It is not surprising, then, that research is showing that not all LDLs are "bad" (or maybe as bad) in terms of cardiovascular risk. There appear to be "good" and "bad" LDLs based on particle size.

The larger LDLs are called "fluffy" or "buoyant" and are full of cholesterol. They are like abundantly loaded inflatable (remember, "buoyant") barges which float down the bloodstream throughout the body to dock at the places where cholesterol is needed.

As the cholesterol cargo is delivered, the LDL barge shrinks until it becomes a small particle LDL. This is basically a depleted LDL.

Herein lies the problem. The small particle LDLs are more prone to oxidization and enzymatic damage, which makes them not useful, and subject to absorption by macrophages, a form of white blood cell. This is the first step in the formation of lesions in the arteries. Because of their smaller size, this type of LDL is more easily able to penetrate the endothelial lining of the arteries to do damage.

For those small particle LDLs which are not damaged, however, their usefulness is not over. This depleted LDL can be recycled by getting reloaded with cholesterol back into its larger, fluffier form. LDLs can be recharged both by the liver and by the HDLs.

fig. 5

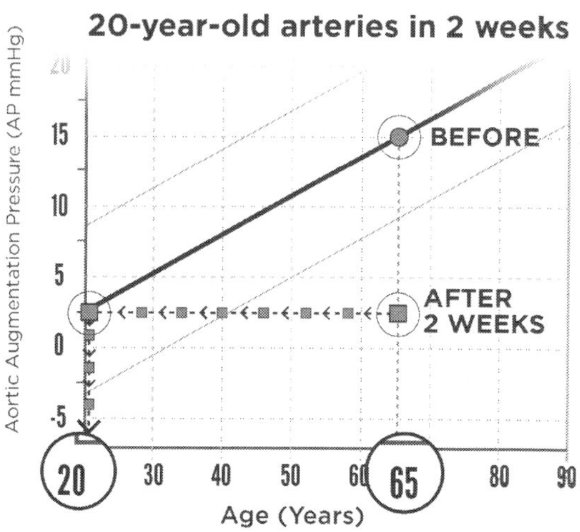

Measurements of arterial stiffness are compared to normal (solid line) for each age. This chart of a 65-year-old male in our study shows how the BalancePoint diet increased the elasticity of his arteries, which started coincidentally like those of a 65-year-old's (people often measure much older than their age), to ones like a 20-year-old's.

HDL reverse transport

The body calls on another type of lipoprotein, the high-density HDL carriers, to collect and scavenge any of the no longer useful cholesterol. They pick up cholesterol from white blood cells called macrophages, which have absorbed and broken down LDLs (phagocytes) for transporting them back to the liver and for re-charging the LDLs. This is called reverse transport. If we see high numbers of HDL in someone, it generally means a lower risk for heart attack due to HDL availability for this reverse transport mechanism.

Eating smaller amounts of protein seems to ramp up production of HDL, or "good cholesterol" particles, and the scavenging of the harmful products depleted of their useful cholesterol. For those who have participated in our diet, and strictly adhered to a low-protein regimen, increases in HDL levels are even more significant. Although we are still collecting data to explore the theory, we believe that this could be because the body, short on protein from external sources, is looking to LDLs (made up of both fat and protein) as a source. To break those LDLs down and extract the needed protein, it primes the pump to make more HDLs.

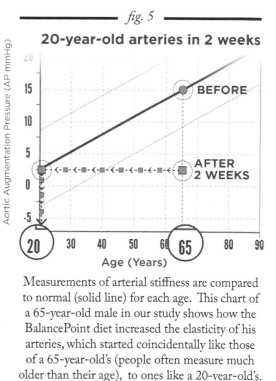

CHAPTER 6
Fight fat with fat

The key to the BalancePoint approach is to re-balance the biochemistry in our body so that our metabolism can work at its best, in the way our genome or body "blueprint" wants it to.

And what does our genome prefer in terms of fat in our food? "Low Fat" has been the mantra for years, and back when I started the BalancePoint program, I raised many a doctor or nutritionist's eyebrow of by explaining that my formula used more than 65% fat content. The "low fat" dictum has been deeply ingrained in our minds, but there is no real scientific evidence supporting the low fat approach. Instead, there seems to have been a "guilt by association" attached to fat—if you want to stop storing fat in your body do not keep putting it in.

EVEN GREAT ATHLETES CAN HAVE HIGH CHOLESTEROL

John Stearns is a former NY Mets All-star and is now a coach with a professional baseball team. Despite working out for hours each day and following a healthy diet, he still had high cholesterol. He tried the BalancePoint protocol at age 57 and reduced his "bad" LDL cholesterol by 64 mg/dl, lost weight and decreased inflammation in his arteries.

However, the genome seems tuned to a high-fat intake. Both our data, and some studies of populations eating this type of diet, appear to support this counter-intuitive approach.

We adapted to a high-fat diet during the long cold periods of our evolutionary history, when fruits and vegetables were not available for large numbers of people. The high levels of fat came from animal fat. Even today, if you look at the Inuit (Eskimo) populations, heart disease was not present when they ate their traditional diet of 85% fat, 15% protein and 0% carbohydrates. In the last couple of generations, after being introduced to our fast-carbohydrate diet, diabetes and obesity are starting to appear in high rates. I have an enduring image of Inuit seal hunters sitting across from me in our extra-long wooden rowboat, floating by an iceberg, while they pulled out a tin of Hudson Bay Company scones for a snack.

The BalancePoint protocol's effectiveness in dramatically reducing cholesterol appears to be directly related to its use of high amounts of fat. If you remember from my description in Chapter 2 of how I developed the diet, my goal is to shift the body's metabolism. We want to switch our bodies to fat or lipid metabolism and we use a lipid-dominant diet to do it. Let me explain.

In our beloved grains we find two major problems: one is the too-fast absorption of carbohydrates and the other is the inflammatory factor in them

Generally speaking, the common American diet, and actually most of the civilized world, is very high in carbohydrates. Think of our traditional staples—bread, potatoes, cereal, pasta... all carbohydrate-dense foods. Where there is agriculture in the world, grains are the dominant staple, whether "staff of life" wheat or rice.

So, what we are doing is something quite unorthodox. With BalancePoint, we are changing the staple, the source of calories, from carbohydrates to lipids. It is a high number— a minimum of 65% to 70% of the calories comes from fats.

But they are "good fats," as some like to say. So you find yourself eating olive oil (in quantities you never imagined yourself consuming), mono-unsaturated oils, avocados, nuts, fish oil tablets—all generally known to be "healthy" fats and a combination of important Omega 3 and Omega 6 elements. Most people do not realize that Omega 3 comes in different forms and all are not of the same benefit to us. Vegetable Omega 3, such as found in flax seeds, is a shorter chain and cannot be used by the body so you need Omega 3 from fish sources.

Let us talk for a moment about the type of fats. We do not know if saturated fats are a problem so we have just made it a part of our plan to use

The end result of BalancePoint's nutritional shift is not only dramatically improved numbers on the lipid panel—such as cholesterol, triglycerides, amount of small particle LDLs—at the doctor's office. By addressing the root of the problem, chronic inflammation, BalancePoint is producing better numbers for people on a whole series of cardiometabolic biomarkers, including abdominal obesity, elevated blood pressure, insulin resistance or glucose intolerance.

what we know to be the healthiest of the fats, which are the mono-unsaturated fats. In any case, we would never use a trans-fat, which is a manufactured fat.

I suspect, however, that other than trans-fats, we will find the type of oil or fat may not be as critical when you are making oils the staple as in the BalancePoint protocol. It may actually not matter whether someone eats more or less amounts of saturated fats as long as there are enough monounsaturated fats in their diet (if you do not get enough monounsaturated fats you can get faulty polymer formations in the heart which increase the risk of heart failure). We may find that certain animal or vegetable fats may be used interchangeably and still achieve rapid reduction of LDL cholesterol. The reason is that once the body's fat-burning metabolism gets cranked up and running with our diet mechanism, the fats are being burned rather than being deposited in the tissue. I have a hunch that further research will prove pork fat to be as effective as olive oil when used according to the BalancePoint formula!

Volunteers?

Shifting metabolism to keep fats burning

So why do we want to switch the metabolism from a carbohydrate one to a lipid or fat one? When you have carbohydrates in the body, they get preferential treatment as a source of energy because they are harder to store. As a result, fats do not get burned—they get stored.

The reason has to do with insulin levels. When you have a lot of carbohydrates that are digested too quickly, such as sugars and starches like potatoes and grains (which are readily converted to sugars) you get what is known as a glycemic spike. It is part of a spike-and-crash cycle of blood sugar levels.

The crash of blood sugar levels is what we experience when exercising as "hitting the wall", and if it is too severe, it is known as hypoglycemia, as we all have experienced when there is a feverish drive to find a doughnut!

Too much sugar can damage, among other things, our red blood cells, and the hormone insulin is used to manage sugar or glucose levels. It does so by directing the liver to convert the excess sugars into a simple fat known as triglycerides. Elevated levels of triglycerides indicate a diet high in rapidly absorbed carbohydrates, and are one of the indicators of metabolic syndrome. So a spike in glucose causes a correlating spike of insulin in the body.

Our goal then is to keep insulin levels low. The spike and crash cycles described above contribute to insulin insensitivity. The body at first cannot sense how much insulin it is producing and makes too much, but then gets to a point where it loses the ability to make it. This is what we call Type 2 Diabetes. Diabetes is a very serious disease for which eye problems, kidney

"Continuous lipid metabolism… to grind up and eat bad cholesterol"

failure, dialysis and even leg amputations are too real a possibility these days. The CDC reports that in 18 states diabetes cases have doubled in the last 15 years. The disease now affects over 8% of Americans.

An equally important reason to keep insulin levels low has to do with the role of insulin in controlling the movement of fat into and out of cells. High levels of insulin inhibit the flow of fat out of cells so that it cannot be metabolized or burned off.

From this discussion, you can see why conditions like obesity and fatty liver are often related to excessive levels of high-glycemic foods and resulting elevated glucose and triglyceride levels.

So the bottom line is that when the body is in carbohydrate metabolism, the metabolism of lipids—the burning off of fats—is shut down so that fats can be stored for later use. Going into storage mode is probably the reason for the problem of raised levels of cholesterol, which, you will remember, is a lipid. That is why I set out to start and keep the lipid-burners on.

To do this requires resetting the metabolic pathway. When fats instead of carbohydrates become the staple to provide energy to the cells, the body cranks up its lipid metabolism. The enzymes needed to metabolize fats for energy also metabolize cholesterol lipoproteins, the LDLs, in the system. So by being in lipid metabolism, not only is fat burned, but also the surplus or unneeded cholesterol as well.

It is this same lipid metabolism that, in spite of the notion of consuming large amounts of fat, has the unexpected effect of making weight loss easier. The reason is self-explanatory. You are already in fat metabolism, and your metabolic pathways are set to keep the fat burners running continuously. Part IV, "Beating the hunger games—weight loss easier with BalancePoint," offers a more detailed discussion on how our diet makes losing weight easier than traditional diets.

So, for many people high fat and lipid metabolism not only equals rapid cholesterol reduction. It can also bring significant weight loss, and the good thing is that you can control it. And, as we keep reminding BalancePoint participants and doctors, you do not have to lose weight if you do not want to and you will still be able to see your cholesterol numbers plummet in two weeks.

I've gone up and down and gained and lost over 300 pounds total over my lifetime trying every diet around. This is the first time I've lost weight—70 pounds—and maintained it. It's such a pleasure not feeling hungry or starving.

My fibromyalgia is much better. I'll have a little flare-up once in a while due to stress. My Rosacea is gone and my hair is thicker and healthy for the first time in my life. (Unfortunately, these improvements didn't come back in my 20's, when I could have really used them!) These are all major improvements in my eye because they are all symptoms of larger health improvements.

I'm astonished at how it's amazing to me how you don't realize how many ailments you're living with until they're gone.

Sandra M., Age 64

CHAPTER 7

Targeting the real villains

Not all LDLs are created equal. The large, fluffy ones are essential for cell repair and the small particle ones have delivered a part of their cholesterol load and now, being cholesterol-depleted, are the ones that do the most damage.

We focus on these small particle LDLs because of the significant link between this particular sub-type of LDL and a greater risk of atherosclerosis. Atherosclerosis, also known colloquially as hardening of the arteries, is the leading cause of strokes, heart attacks, and most forms of cardiovascular disease. It can begin in adolescence, or even earlier, and is usually not detected. The first symptom is often a heart attack, or in up to one-third of patients, sudden death. So more attention is now paid to the size of the LDL particle.

When you get your standard blood test or lipid panel, it does not give this detail. More sophisticated tests (using either NMR, nuclear magnetic resonance, or centrifugal technology) differentiate between the number of large "fluffy" LDLs versus small particle LDLs. Recent studies show that measuring the concentration of small particle LDLs is a more accurate predictor of the risk associated with LDLs in general.

So imagine two scenarios. One is a person who believes he is "safe" because he has a low

GOLD-MEDAL PERFORMANCE

The Tour of the Gila is a 5-day bicycle race that is known as one of the toughest amateur stage races in North America. In 2007, then 29-year-old Brian Loflin placed 37th overall. Then he went on BalancePoint. In the 2008 race, he placed 1st overall!

"The BalancePoint eating plan allowed me to decrease my body fat percentage by eating in a healthy manner. I managed to drop 10 to 11 lbs before the race. My energy levels increased and the decrease in weight allowed my power to weight ratio to increase. The one draw back I would say is that during the first week of the eating plan, my body had to adjust and my training suffered; however after my body was used to the eating style and Binx modified my protein intake slightly, is when I started to feel better and recover from training. Overall, I would say the eating style allowed my body to become a fine-tuned machine which improved my racing."

LDL count. But we find out it is made up of all small particle LDLs. The other is someone with a much higher LDL count, but with a large percentage of the LDLs being the more benign, large fluffy type. The first indicates significantly greater risk. However, most of us would not know that because we are trained to look simply at the total count of LDLs, whether large or small sized.

We generally do not know the specific make-up of our LDLs because the more refined tests are expensive and not commonly available. Doctors do not normally order them unless someone is at high risk. Also, the standard treatment for high LDLs has been drugs, which lower the amount of all types of LDLs.

The very common cholesterol-lowering drugs called statins have been a miracle solution for many people with high risk factors for heart disease. They are in fact the most prescribed drug in the world. As with many strong medications, they are not without their own risks. If we look at their mechanism, we get a clue why. Statins lower LDL levels by suppressing their production in the liver. There is a cascade effect. The LDLs emerging from the liver are large, fluffy ones and, as we have explained, they become depleted of their cholesterol and end up as small particle LDLs. By reducing their number, there are less LDLs in total to be converted into small particle LDLs. So, by default, there are less small particle LDLs. This problem, though, is that large fluffy LDLs are necessary for cell and muscle repair, perhaps explaining the sometimes side effect of muscle cramps or paralysis and memory loss when taking statins.

When we started using the more complex, broad-spectrum cholesterol tests, we made an intriguing discovery: the BalancePoint protocol almost always significantly reduces the number of small particle LDLs. The number of beneficial large, fluffy LDLs are hardly reduced at all.

So BalancePoint appears to target the most problematic type of LDLs, while leaving the beneficial ones to continue their work.

No drug therapy has been shown to accomplish this. Now that we are providing for the first time a way to directly diminish the levels of small particle LDLs, we expect that more efforts will be made to make available on a wider basis the tests to measure them.

What this means is that BalancePoint is not "fixing" LDLs—we are allowing the body to bring the systems back into proper operation. This effect of disposing of only these no longer useful forms of, and not all, LDLs was also one of my earliest clues that what BalancePoint does is prompt the body to heal itself.

Why small particle LDLs cause problems

So why does the body try to minimize these small particle LDLs?

If the wall of the artery is inflamed, then the small particle LDLs can slip through, just as in a sieve. Small particle LDLs are much more prone to oxidation. Our typical diets today tend to be high in free radicals, which cause oxidation, a damaging process that ends the LDLs' usefulness as a cholesterol transporter and makes them targets for absorption by macrophages. This leads to the development of lesions or plaque in the arteries.

(The body deposits calcium over their surface to armor these lesions, much like a scab over a wound, and this is what increasingly popular calcium scans measure. The calcium is not the plaque we are talking about.)

With the BalancePoint concepts I have learned, I now seem to be able to control aspects of my weight and cardiovascular health that I had previously felt were largely out of my control. I lost more than 15 pounds and in just two weeks, the stiffness of my arteries improved from the equivalent of a 90-year-old to that of a 40-year-old, and my blood pressure dropped from 155/130 to 120/80. I have not regained any of the weight I have lost. Many aspects of the food protocol now seem quite natural to me.

J.P., Age 50

There are basically three ways in which the lesions or plaque can cause problems. One is that they cause the endothelial wall to swell around them, making the opening of the artery smaller. This is called stenosis. Blood flow is restricted, closing off the vessel to different degrees, and because the blood supply is limited, it results in a lack of energy and symptoms of angina pain in the chest or other pain such as in the legs. Angioplasty techniques and insertion of stints were popular treatments but are now losing favor as their effectiveness is being questioned.

Another effect of plaque is that the lesions can break open like a boil does.

It releases in a sudden burst a lot of foreign material into the bloodstream. The cardiovascular system's reaction is to shut down and cut off circulation. This is a myocardial infarction, known commonly as a heart attack.

A third possibility is that waxy pieces of the plaque can break loose, get caught in an artery and plug the flow to certain areas of the brain, where the pieces lodge. This is what happens with a stroke.

And it all starts with inflammation.

BalancePoint appears to target the most problematic type of LDLs, while leaving the beneficial ones to continue their work. No drug therapy has been shown to accomplish this.

CHAPTER 8

Lower inflammation in days

Yes, BalancePoint quickly corrects cholesterol levels and reduces the amount of the most dangerous form of LDLs, the small particle-size ones. But the really exciting news is that BalancePoint quickly reduces chronic inflammation in the body.

In fact, the importance of Balance Point's ability to manage cholesterol levels with diet and no drugs is dwarfed by its anti-inflammatory power. You may have picked up this book simply because you were told by your doctor to reduce your cholesterol numbers. By going on the BalancePoint protocol, however, the benefits will go beyond what you and your doctor may be expecting.

You will be getting to the source of not only cholesterol imbalance but many other ailments in the body—chronic inflammation. So you will find that biomarkers for other conditions that you may have never thought of as related to high cholesterol will show significant improvement. Incidentally, cholesterol-lowering drugs with their highly targeted approach do not achieve this same overall effect.

Reducing chronic inflammation has huge benefits. It opens the way to not just weakening or even healing its effects, but doing so very rapidly.

Yes, BalancePoint quickly corrects cholesterol levels... But the really exciting news is that BalancePoint quickly reduces chronic inflammation in the body.

Secondary to that, it appears that all of the inflammatory diseases, **not only osteoarthritis and allergies, but also asthma and even susceptibility to cancer, can be notably reduced. Newest medical and scientific understanding of inflammation suggests**

that it is at the root of a whole series of aging-related disease. Not only heart disease, but also diabetes, metabolic syndrome, high blood pressure, osteoarthritis, Alzheimer's disease, as well as many non age-related diseases including cancer, obesity, acne, and depression are now being linked to chronic inflammation in the body.

The American Academy of Periodontology convened a conference in 2008 which went beyond gum disease and drew together opinion leaders in several "major diseases and the inflammatory mechanisms that seem to underlie and unify all of these diseases."

Those are the words of Dr. Thomas Van Dyke, Boston University, who published the resulting paper, "Inflammation and Periodontal Diseases: A Reappraisal" in August 2008. Dr. Van Dyke notes that there has been a very recent "explosion of scientific knowledge on inflammation and chronic disease of aging." He refers to the "new knowledge of inflammation" and how "inflammation is now known to play a critical role in diseases that are not usually classified as inflammatory disease, such as cardiovascular disease and Alzheimer's disease." (I bring attention to this paper because it introduces a whole series of important new scientific research presented at this conference on inflammatory-related diseases.)

How inflammation plays this underlying role in all these disorders is a fascinating question with many answers. In the case of allergies, for instance, I suspect there seems to be a synergistic effect with certain pollens and other irritants such that if there is no chronic inflammation present, there may not be the trigger to activate the allergic reaction.

As a side point, looking at inflammation as a key to understanding cancer is probably a new concept for most of us. Basically, the concept proposes that it is chronic inflammation, rather than mutant cells running amok, which contribute to the cause of cancer. In the normal healing process, the body tries to induce growth of cells to fix the problem. As explained later, inflammation is a natural response in the body to call for repair teams. Once the job is done, the inflammation normally goes away and the healing goes through its natural sequence of events. However, when the inflammatory state lasts too long the natural healing process is sabotaged or subverted. This chronic inflammation may instead promote malignant and uncontrolled growth of cells. This new theory is explained in laymen's terms in a 2007 *Scientific American* article called, "The Malignant Flame":

"As some researchers have described the malignant state: genetic damage is the match that lights the fire, and inflammation is the fuel that feeds it."

Accordingly, the article offers this food for thought: "This new view implies that rooting out every last cancer cell in the body might not be necessary. Anti-inflammatory cancer therapy instead would prevent premalignant cells from turning fully cancerous or would impede an existing tumor from spreading to distant sites in the body."

This approach of using anti-inflammatory therapy could well work for a number of diseases, in particular age-related chronic conditions, we have talked about throughout the book.

The link between inflammation and heart disease was an early revelation with BalancePoint results. The role of inflammation, and the effectiveness of our BalancePoint protocol in alleviating its damage, first came to light with our first group of diet participants over six years ago. We continue to see that a reduction of inflammation helps improve a whole series of risk factors for a wide range of cardiometabolic and other health conditions. You can see this on fig. 1 in Part I.

You will see that BalancePoint's fast-acting anti-inflammatory effect includes two lines of attack:

• Removal of pro-inflammatory triggers and

• Use of what leading edge medical researchers are calling "inflammatory terminators."

So let us look more closely on how BalancePoint is giving new understanding of the connection between high cholesterol and other cardiometabolic risk factors and inflammation.

"The body is a piece of incredible natural engineering. In most cases, it is designed to operate without having to take drugs every day."

CHAPTER 9

Getting to the root of heart and metabolic diseases

Inflammation is a natural process that the body goes through in response to an emergency such as an injury or infection. It is a call to arms that the body sends out through chemical and neurological messengers for marshalling the body's defensive systems. The swelling from the inflammation expands the cells around the wound or invader to provide openings for the white blood cell "soldiers", called macrophages, to rush in more easily to take over the intruders. The tissue get damaged in the process, so a second call goes out for the repair crew, namely cholesterol, which brings restorative material to the site.

In a person who does not have chronic inflammation, the inflammation then dies down fairly quickly and the normal healing process takes over.

Chronic inflammation, on the other hand, is like having troops stay on alert all the time. Fatigue sets in and problems start to arise.

Inflammation lets small particle LDLs in to do their dirty work

Cardiovascular disease, high cholesterol, or other metabolic diseases are a sign that there is chronic inflammation present. These cardiometabolic problems are due to a number of factors, including diet, environmental conditions, stress, and inactivity. The primary cause, though, is diet.

Certain foods induce an inflammatory condition which can often be seen right away in the intestines—and also in the vascular system. The inflammation causes the endothelial walls of the arteries to swell, becoming rough and open. Think of when your skin gets a rash or gets inflamed and, same thing, it becomes swollen or vulnerable and is much more prone to getting an infection or a secondary problem. That is also true in our arteries.

When the endothelial walls open up, they become far more permeable. LDLs have been summoned there to provide cholesterol for repair. However, the depleted small particle LDLs, because of their size, slip easily through the "sieve" of the inflammation-damaged endothelial wall. They build up behind the wall, forming lesions which eventually can become quite extensive. The plaque builds up causing narrowing of the arteries, leading to angina and vascular flow problems, and the plaque itself can break away or rupture, leading to a stroke or heart attack, as we described earlier.

And all these potentially debilitating or fatal conditions start with inflammation. The prevailing medical thinking is that the lesion and plaque build up from LDL cholesterol causes the inflammation in the arteries, leading to atherosclerosis. I, however, believe our evidence gives a different view: that it is the other way around, and it is inflammation which is the root problem and opens the walls of arteries to allow the LDLs in to do the damage.

In addition, as explained at the end of this chapter, I suspect that if you did not have inflammation your levels of cholesterol would not really be that much of a factor, and you would not get heart disease.

Our tests and evidence of inflammation reduction

The good news is the BalancePoint dietary protocol can cure inflammatory conditions within days. We can see this from before-and-after clinical tests of the stiffness of arteries.

In testing our diet participants, we have noted that people who have extremely stiff arteries, or essentially significant inflammation in their cardiovascular system, generally have high levels of cholesterol. It makes sense. Inflammation in the body puts out a call for repair and for the front line of defense. And that includes a call for cholesterol, which is essential for cell repair.

"It was assumed that cholesterol triggered the inflammation. Our observations pointed me in the opposite direction."

INFLAMMATION → CHOLESTEROL

Not all calories are created equal. High amounts of fat will leave you feeling much more satisfied and less hungry.

Our studies lead us to believe that a high percentage of the population harbors this type of inflammation, but most of us at a low chronic level. This low-level chronic inflammation in our blood vessels can be seen as one of the factors in developing stiff arteries.

Inflammation causes swelling the walls of the artery, which become thicker and therefore stiffer. To measure the stiffness we use a simple, non-invasive test which measures what we could call "internal blood pressure" of our arteries. It gives a more sophisticated and accurate reading of the health of our vessels than what is given from the traditional cuff we put around our arms. A normal reading from the cuff might not reveal how rigid the arteries actually are. (There is probably a good chance that stiffness of the arteries had not been measured in the case of some high-profile celebrities needing heart surgery or even suddenly dying when other high risk factors were not evident.)

To do this test, a pressure transducer probe shaped like a pen is placed on top of your wrist at a pulse point to get a waveform reading. It then measures the reflective wave of the pulse after it is sent out from the heart, hits a certain spot in the groin where the arteries branch out, and rushes back. If your arteries have the elasticity of something like a balloon, then there is some "give" as the balloon expands, and the reflective wave is slower and smaller. But if the walls of the arteries are rigid then the return wave of the pulse comes back more quickly through the body.

The technology, called sphygmography, has been used mainly in research facilities rather than in medical clinics and its price has not been low enough to encourage widespread use. And, until BalancePoint, it might have been unclear to doctors how to treat high readings showing a stiff vascular system in a patient.

Stiff arteries become more elastic in days on BalancePoint

Since most over weight people are carbohydrate burners they do not have well-developed lipid burning metabolism, and to be able to actually lose weight, you have to burn fat to burn off body fat.

We have noted that almost everyone shows a significant drop in this arterial stiffness measurement after going on the BalancePoint two-week protocol. The numbers are correlated to what would be expected for someone at a given age. This is called an age-equivalent database. Our tests show that the arterial stiffness of people on the BalancePoint diet drops rapidly in even a few days and then continues to drop at a slower rate until they gain the elasticity of a much younger individual.

It is not unusual to see our people drop thirty or forty years in their age equivalency of their vascular system. So someone whose arterial stiffness is equivalent to that of a 100-year-old (which can easily happen with those showing high cholesterol combined with other cardiometabolic conditions) can drop to that of a 60-year-old, or a 50-year-old, and in many cases will at the end of BalancePoint's two-week program show arteries like someone in their 20's.

Such spectacular drops in a few days after going on the BalancePoint protocol is not that unusual when the initial reading is high. This reading if taken after someone's been on BalancePoint usually drops to a range closer to what you would expect of a person that age. (Or lower. Even people who already have arteries the same as someone twenty years younger can still produce a decrease of ten or more years.)

Our goal in using this sphygmography measurement is to see what kind of improvement someone shows in their inflammatory condition. Another biomarker more familiar to many is C-Reactive protein, which is being used more and more frequently. It however is an indirect measurement, done through blood tests. Also, some people who have inflammation do not have this protein in their bodies. The sphygmography test measures actual physical reaction so is probably a better indicator of inflammation. However, for people who are unable to come to our facility for assessment, we will be using the C-reactive protein alternative.

Recovery from inflammation a two-phase process

Our experience with the testing of stiffness of the arteries gives us an interesting insight into inflammation. We get significant reductions in inflammation in just days with BalancePoint. From this finding, I suspect that recovery from inflammation is a two-step process.

The first phase comes from reduction of the inflammation itself. We talked about the initial drop we see in arterial stiffness. This is probably due to diminishing of the inflammation level itself since that would be the logical explanation of what could produce such a rapid and dramatic response. So this inflammation can leave the body within a few days.

Or, as another example, almost all the BalancePoint participants who normally have some sort of arthritic pain start to notice a significant improvement in as little as a few days after starting the diet.

We then often see slower improvement occurring over the following months. This is what I see as the second phase of the effects of inflammation, and that concerns the damage done by inflammation.

In the case of the stiff arteries, there is sclerotic damage or hardening of the arteries that involves the build-up of deposits in the arteries. This amounts

BUT THE HEART-HEALTHY PEOPLE IN CRETE EAT BREAD... DON'T THEY?

The Seven Countries Study by Ancel Keys pinpointed Crete as a place with significantly lower heart disease than any of the other Mediterranean countries, including mother country Greece itself. But isn't bread a staple of their diet?

If you go to the core of Crete, you will find people still living the same way they did long ago. People had grandparents living well past 100 years old, and none of them had heart disease. You look at the bearded goat herders and they are energetic and robust, shepherding goats on cliffs so sheer that I do not even know how the goats let alone men got up and down them. In the mountain tavernas you can find menus full of vegetables with Greek names which I had never heard of—all kinds of wild greens that they still gather.

It turns out that they eat very little bread, at least not the kind you would expect. They ate these things called rusks, which are loaves of bread with deep cuts in them so that, after they are baked, they are broken into these big slices of bread put them back in the cooled-off oven to completely dry them out.

So it was a puzzle. It looked like they were eating coarse grain, but our studies showed that even coarse grains raised cholesterol

to injury to the cardiovascular system and could take a year to heal before we see reversal of heart disease.

Similarly, we see people getting rid of symptoms of arthritis in a few days, but the healing from harm done to the body from the actual arthritis could take a long time, or not happen at all.

Sometimes, the damage from a longer, chronic inflammatory state might be just too far along, as in the case of a badly damaged arthritic joint or cancer, for the body to repair itself. But maybe not.

The hope we have is that, in most cases, once the inflammation is brought under control, then the body can work on healing itself and restoring itself to normal.

Lowering inflammation lets cholesterol do its useful work

So the fact that the BalancePoint diet causes the blood vessels to gain back their elasticity is an indication that this chronic inflammation in our body is being reduced. As that happens, the swelling and the thickening of the blood vessels of the endothelial wall decrease and the arteries become much more elastic. With chronic inflammation decreasing, the cardiovascular lining can start to heal and regain its health.

levels. I then came across research on little proteins called lectins that are concentrated in the kernel of the grain. When researchers fed people with very coarse grains and more refined grains that had less of the germ, they actually found a higher incidence of heart disease in those that ate the coarser grains. So it appears that for people who are sensitive to this class of lectins, whole grains are a bad choice. (For people who are not, it is healthier to have the whole grains because it has a lower glycemic index. However, we believe this last group makes up only 10 or 15% of the population.)

And so, that research led me to some new work of Italian researchers who have been analyzing the impact of sourdough fermentation on bread in terms of reducing its glycemic index. They discovered that if you ferment dough for 24 hours instead of the usual 4 or 8 hours, the bread became almost reaction-free for people who had Celiac's disease.

Well, guess what? The Cretans' bread starter sits for a whole week or two fermenting! So…the reason that the rusks do not bother them is probably because of this extra-long fermentation! My guess is that the fermentation process breaks down the lectins (which are apparently causing all these inflammation problems.) The rusks have both the low glycemic index and the coarse grain. And the other thing is that the Cretans do not eat a lot of them. All interesting pieces of the puzzle.

Not surprisingly, blood pressure improves as well.

It has been previously thought that the best line of attack to control high cholesterol is to inhibit the production of cholesterol. That is what statin drugs do.

BalancePoint, however, takes a different approach. What we do is to manage or enhance the production of cholesterol. We lower LDLs by letting cholesterol do its work—in the way it was meant to. BalancePoint gets rid of the inflammation so that the arteries can operate in nice, clean, inflammation-free walls. The routes for the LDL "barges" we spoke about earlier are not blocked. So the LDLs are free to deliver their payloads of cholesterol for useful purposes such as cell repair or bile production, or whatever the body is calling for.

This is a very important point regarding BalancePoint's role in reducing inflammation in the body. Statins do not make inflammation go away like BalancePoint does. The blood test results we get showing a return to balance in the whole cholesterol picture, not just the lowering of one type of LDL, appears to confirm that BalancePoint's anti-inflammatory action is allowing cholesterol to naturally do what it is supposed to do in the body so that it is no longer a problem.

No wonder the traditional dieting process becomes so difficult. You are continually going into starvation mode and your body is screaming at you to get another bagel at any cost!

The link between inflammation and heart disease

Since heart disease is an inflammatory disease we believe this may mean if you have no inflammation, you probably cannot get cardiovascular disease, independent of what your cholesterol levels are. We would be more like the animals who, if there is no damage to the arterial walls, would require extremely high levels of cholesterol to get plaque formation in the arteries.

More research needs to be done to confirm this hypothesis and to better define and understand the arterial stiffness reduction. The fact that a number of different populations around the world, such as people of Crete in the late '50s early '60s, were essentially heart disease free with a diet with some of the attributes of the BalancePoint protocol, coupled with our success in reversing arterial stiffness in many people, helps point to our suggestion that heart disease may very well be optional.

The American Diabetes Association and the American College of Cardiology Foundation have just jointly issued in 2008 a "Consensus Statement" which is earmarked to be an important reference for use in the medical world. This scientific paper describes the contribution of lipoproteins to risk of cardiovascular and metabolic disease and suggests best treatment for managing them. It is an excellently written resource and I encourage all readers of this book to look at it. It includes one particular observation that I found very intriguing in terms of our research.

The authors of this paper point out that in animal studies it takes cholesterol levels more than 800 mg/dL of cholesterol to cause lesion formation unless there is "direct arterial injury." This is a very high number—more than four times the normal level. High cholesterol levels also appear to be necessary for the formation of lesions in humans, where lesion development usually occurs over many decades. However, it takes far less lower levels in humans than for animals for this to happen.

I find the BalancePoint protocol very satisfying and relatively easy to maintain but I do see my need for the olive oil, especially for satisfying hunger. I have lost 35 pounds and feel great. My blood pressure is much more stable and all my heart symptoms of arrhythmia and racing heart are gone. I like to make up a mixture of raw sunflower seeds, pumpkins seeds, and chopped pecans, walnuts, and almonds, which have been soaked overnight in warm water and then baked in an 110° oven for at least 10 hours, to use as either a snack or yogurt topping, depending on what I need—or don't need—to fit my calories and nutrient formula for the day.

Verone C.

I believe that the reason for this lower threshold level in humans is that we do get injury to our arteries. It comes not from what we normally think of as wounds, but from chronic inflammation. Our American diet turns out to be pro-inflammatory to the extent that chronic inflammation is present in a majority of us. Most of us do not exhibit obvious signs of it, yet it is still quietly present with its potential for initiating disease.

In one scenario, this inflammation damages the endothelial wall of the arteries, allowing small particle LDLs to enter, forming lesions leading to heart disease. An unhealthy lipid profile (high total cholesterol and LDL, high triglycerides, low HDL) is a significant risk factor for cardiovascular disease, so improving the profile is important. But, in my view, it is probably less important than eliminating chronic inflammation.

Fortunately, the BalancePoint Diet does both: improves the cholesterol profile and reduces inflammation.

Inflammation requires cholesterol for repair of inflammatory damage. This stimulates LDL production and increases their levels. When the inflammation levels are low, LDLs drop and the need for HDLs drops as well.

As we said in the beginning of this chapter, the problem with our rapidly changing diet and lifestyle is that we are getting outside of the genome's area of expertise. The result is marginal performance and degenerative diseases of aging. **The reason we use the name BalancePoint for the diet is because it is about finding the lifestyle "sweet spot" in the genome. It is the point where nutrition and the foods in our diet, plus activity and stress management, are optimized so that the genome can maintain optimal health. The medical science mission of BalancePoint is to create the food environment in which the largest percentage of people can be successful in finding that health.**

CHAPTER 10

Inflammatory triggers in our food

Some of our favorites are the villains, armed with genetic incompatibility and newly identified poison pill protein

I earlier said the good news is that BalancePoint has the power to lower inflammation, and in just two weeks. The bad news concerns the foods which we are finding to be very pro-inflammatory. Grains, sad to say, are one of the prime culprits. And, unfortunately, it appears to be all, not just some, grains that are guilty.

When some people hear about our "no grains" rule, their response is, "No way. I'd rather take a pill." We all love our grains, which make up most of our traditional "comfort food", but we are learning from the latest science discoveries how most of us do not tolerate grains. And, for those of you aware of gluten sensitivities, who think that avoiding gluten-containing bread and crackers gets you off the hook, sorry. The grains that cause problems include spelt, wheat, oats, corn, rye and rice.

Our clinical evidence shows fast effect of grains

Our first hint about the problematic effect of grains came in some of our earliest research in 2006 when our first group on the two-week BalancePoint Jumpstart Program asked if they could add a few

"I DON'T HAVE A PROBLEM—MY LDLS ARE LOW." BUT, WHEN IS THIS A PROBLEM?

In the early days of BalancePoint, someone came up to me asking if I could do the opposite—raise his LDLs. I had just read a medical research paper linking low LDLs to Celiac disease. Even though he had tested negative for Celiac disease, I suspected otherwise. After going on BalancePoint, his LDLs went up and he said his mood swings, which he had had all his life, went away. And medical tests have confirmed he is a Celiac. Now, whenever people come to us saying they have "very low" LDL numbers and their cholesterol profiles also reveal an accompanying low level of HDLs, our first suspicion is that they may be a Celiac. After going on BalancePoint, these people find a remarkable change in not only their cholesterol numbers, but also in their Celiac symptoms because it is an ideal diet for Celiacs.

foods like meat and grains back in their diet. The group had seen dramatic, 40-50 mg/dl reductions in their LDL. Now they wanted to see if they could maintain them with a more lenient protocol. Each participant was allowed to add one food back into the diet while maintaining the proper ratio of fat, protein and carbohydrates. The re-introduced foods included brown rice, Irish-cut whole grain oatmeal, 100% whole-wheat coarse-grain bread—all the "healthiest" variations of grains we are told to eat. After a couple weeks we tested everyone's cholesterol.

The results were interesting. Adding back red meat only raised LDL a few points. Adding grains, however, caused newly-lowered LDL levels to shoot back up about 50% higher.

We wondered whether it was simply the high glycemic nature of grains that was the problem, or if there was some unique aspect of these monocot plants, which are basically grasses, that was raising back the LDL levels we had just dramatically brought down. So for the time being we referred to it as "the grain factor," and actually labeled it that way in our patent application for the diet.

It got even more interesting when we added the sphygmograph to our standard tests. When people ate grains, we could see an immediate and significant increase in stiffness in their arteries. We would see augmentation pressure climb the next day. Then, over the next two or three days,

Lectin proteins [are like] sticks of super glue... For most of us—we estimate from our BalancePoint observations as many as 80% or so—these lectins do get into our vessels. And when they do, they probably damage the endothelial wall of the arteries to cause inflammation... and the arterial system gets stiffer.

augmentation pressure would drop down to its pre-grain level—as long as these people stayed away from grains.

And then the aches and pains that people reported going away on BalancePoint returned when they tried eating grains again. It soon came to be a strong, predictable tie-in. It reminded me of the suspected connection between recurrent childhood ear infections and low-level chronic inflammation caused by milk and grains.

At first I wondered whether the inflammatory trigger we were witnessing involved a common protein in grains known as gluten. You have probably noticed increasing supermarket shelf space given to "gluten-free" products, or perhaps you know someone with Celiac disease, which is an intolerance of gluten. Gluten does intestinal damage and Celiac disease can be a very serious disorder. For some people it is totally debilitating, involving several organs. Others have a mild form, and some have it in a silent form with almost invisible symptoms. In the past, tests for Celiac disease have produced false negatives but tests developed in the past couple of years are proving more accurate and it is now thought that a greater percentage of the population than we realized are victims of Celiac disease.

However, many of the grains that made blood pressure shoot up and arteries grow stiffer in our

THE MALNUTRITION OF CIVILIZATION

Our clever minds
develop faster than our bodies

Our diet has slowly evolved over the past 50 million years. During temperate and warm periods, we adapted to a diet of foliage, fruit, insects, nuts, eggs, and very small animals. During cold and ice age periods we out of necessity turned to animals with high fat content. So we became well adapted to this broad range of foods, but our brains had the inclination to find the foods with the highest density of calories possible.

Anthropologist Katherine Milton discovered that the bigger the brain the more skill the primates had at know when, as in seasons, and where, as in which trees, fruit or nuts could be found. This cleverness in our human brains started getting ahead of evolution. 10,000 years ago, with the drive for finding calorie-dense foods, we discovered grains, and the relatively complicated ways to be able to use them (harvesting, grinding, cooking—until then all foods were raw).

This was the start of agriculture. We embraced our new diets quickly, but our bodies haven't adapted as fast as our minds could.

We previously had the discernment to guide us to being very selective of what foliage to eat, how much to eat, when to seek out fruit or maybe a little fish or animal food for protein, or large amounts of fat and organ meat in the periods of severe cold.

Once agriculture made it easy to find food, we started to lose this subtle sense, and we began processing foods in order to satisfy cravings for the taste of pure sugar or white flour and rice. We also became wealthier to pay for the increased cost of processing, and we see today how in newly developing countries the previous luxury of feast foods are now available on a daily basis.

We lost the cues to avoid becoming overweight and not fall victim to associated diseases of our cardiovascular and metabolic systems.

All is not bleak—it would be if we did not make changes. Disorders like heart disease and stroke, diabetes, and metabolic syndrome will bankrupt our health systems if we do not act. We now understand how problematic our eating habits have become, a case of malnutrition of civilization. Our mission is to help change that.

- Binx Selby 2006

BalancePoint participants did not contain gluten. So, my speculation was that our culprit might be a protein in grains that was similar, but slightly different, from gluten.

For a year we referred to this mysterious inflammatory property as a "factor" in grains. Then one day I finally had a name for it—a protein called a lectin.

"Poisin pill" protects grains from predators... including us

The presentation of lectins as a possible culprit came in a roundabout way A small news item in *Science* was brought to my attention by a close friend, who had been suffering through a year's worth of lunch conversations dominated by my enthusiastic reports on the latest BalancePoint research developments. The news item reported on how Swedish researchers found that the "Paleolithic" diet free of grains and dairy products performed better than the often-recommended Mediterranean diet for lowering blood sugar in diabetics.

The focus of that study was on the effect of diet on glucose levels and tolerance. But the fact that a diet similar to that of our pre-agriculture ancestors, who ate no grains, worked better for a metabolic disorder than the Mediterranean diet, which includes a lot of grains, piqued my curiosity. This led me to other research papers written by this group of Swedish researchers based out of Lund University. It turns out that a couple years previously, they had published a paper discussing a class of proteins common in grains and beans called lectins. This paper laid out a hypothesis about the effect of lectins on insulin resistance and obesity. It got me thinking about how we at BalancePoint were getting not just inflammation but also higher LDL counts—a link to metabolic dysfunction—from grains.

Aha! This was exactly what I was looking for—a possible identification of the "factor" that was shooting up our LDL levels and causing the rapid increase in stiffness in the arteries.

So what are these lectins? They are small, biologically active proteins and are found in all kinds of foods. They bind reversibly to specific sugar structures and act almost like a hormone.

Different kinds of lectins, each with their unique biochemical properties, appear in different classes of plants. There is a subclass of lectins found only in grass-like grains often referred to as cereals. These particular kind of lectins are concentrated in the kernels of the wheat, oats, barley, corn, or other monocot plants. The lectins do not seem to have any biological function in the metabolism of the grain. What is more, the lectins appear to function as a sort of biocide "poison pill" or protector against getting eaten. When predators eat the grain kernels, the lectins attack and knock out various metabolic systems and regulatory systems.

What happens if humans are the predators? Lectins are adept at sticking to certain polysaccharides, or sugar structures, in animals, of which we are one. Interestingly, they do not stick to plant polysaccharides.

They are sort of like sticks of super glue which attach only to specific sites in our bodies. In fact, they are used in blood typing for this reason. There is a lectin that is very specific to type A blood, and if it coagulates and aggregates into little clumps when you put a drop of it in the blood sample, you know that it is type A.

Hormones operate by attaching to certain sites in the body and sending signals for a particular response. Lectins also act this way, and in Part IV, we will look at how lectins throw off our hormonal balance to promote obesity.

But in terms of possible inflammatory action, we need to look at a lectin called WGA (wheat germ agglutinin). WGA is tied to aggregation, which is the pulling together of the tissue it has stuck to, whether it is intestinal lining or the endothelial wall of the arteries. Because of the "glue" effect of the lectins, when this lining moves, as it does in normal operation, it gets torn.

These lectins are difficult for the body to resist. They are very good at surviving the digestive process without getting broken down and they are clever at being able to get transported into the blood system. This problem does not occur for everyone, as some people appear to have a resistance to the lectins getting into the bloodstream. But for most of us—we estimate from our BalancePoint observations as many as 80% or so—these lectins do get into our vessels.

Avoiding gluten-containing bread and crackers [does not get] you off the hook, sorry

And when they do, they probably damage the endothelial wall of the arteries to cause inflammation. When we constantly eat the grains containing these troublesome lectins, the endothelial wall becomes increasingly vulnerable and inflamed and the arterial system gets stiffer. Our resistance to cholesterol penetration decreases and the small particle LDLs can penetrate into the artery. This causes lesions and plaque formation, the onset of arterial-sclerotic cardiovascular disease.

The idea that grains somehow contribute to these diseases seems to make a lot of sense when you consider that these disorders have been getting more and more prevalent as we eat more and more snack and preprocessed foods which are very much grain-based.

As part of the roundabout process I talked about earlier leading me to lectins, a journalist who recently came to do a radio interview of me happened to know the evolutionary nutritionist Loren Cordain. Dr. Cordain is a professor at Colorado State University, less than two hours away from where I was living in Boulder, so we hopped into the car to go meet him. The author of *The Paleo Diet*, he proposes that the diet from our hunter-gatherer days may be more closely aligned to what our genes still prefer, and is working on theories of the effect of lectins and how they get into the bloodstream. He therefore calls grains, "the two-edged sword"—a boon to the development of civilization but a calamity to our metabolic systems.

Why are almost all of us vulnerable to lectins?

The answer might lie in our evolutionary history. Grains, milk products, and beans are a number of foods which did not make it into the human diet until the invention of agriculture. That was 10,000 years or about 300 generations ago.

From the perspective of population growth necessitating efficiency of production, winter storage and protection against famine, agriculture was a boon for us. It enabled sedentary existence and allowed us to create dense cities. We could grow enough food to support a large population in a small area, and the food could keep over the seasons. It was an ideal situation in many ways and we could rely on calorie-dense grains as our food staple.

On the other hand, grains became our first "processed" food. Anthropologists like Katherine Milton make the case that the rapid success and adoption of grains in our human diet was too speedy for what we could genetically adapt to. Archaeological records of teeth and bones of our ancestors show that

LOSING BELLY FAT

With our two-week Jumpstart program, often people already see the difference in the size of their "paunch"—which doctors are now viewing as a sign of one of greatest risk factors for heart and metabolic disease. A 2008 German study published in The New England Journal of Medicine, found that excess fat around the abdomen nearly doubled a person's risk of death from a variety of diseases, including cancer, stroke and cardiovascular disease.

The problem is that this fat acts differently than the fat we collect around our arms or thighs. Unlike that type of fat which sits around waiting to be burned as energy, this more harmful fat around the waist is biologically active and produces hormones and chemicals which cause inflammation throughout the body.

Fat deposits in the liver, increased cholesterol, triglycerides and blood pressure, and vulnerability to diabetes are some of the serious consequences. A waist circumference of over 36 inches for women and over 40 inches for men is now considered a medical call for action.

Fortunately, BalancePoint has proven very effective at removing this dangerous fat. And it is worthy to note that when we shift people into fat-burning metabolism we target fat deposits around the waist, and the old theory of having to do special stomach-flattening exercises doesn't hold anymore (but daily exercise and physical activity are still important for basic health reasons.)

heart disease and periodontal disease do not appear until grains appeared.

Ten thousand years is only a split-second in our 50 million years of evolutionary history as primates. It is not enough time for our genome to adapt. I am sure that early on there was some adaptation that happened rapidly in the human population as people who had serious intolerance died off. Because mild chronic inflammation creates degenerative conditions, such as arthritis and heart disease, that do not start showing up until mid life, after the reproductive years, it has much less impact on the natural selection process. Each generation continues to bear children. In fact, we had more children once we could rely on agriculture, because we could support larger families. (We needed them to work in the grain fields!) The traits for tolerance of grains were not selected out as strongly as roadblocks in our evolution, and the adaptation for grains has been the kind of development that is a very slow process.

So, in our beloved grains we find two major problems: one is the too-fast absorption of carbohydrates and the other is the inflammatory factor in them.

Milk another comfort food that brings discomfort

Fresh milk products are also proving to be pro-inflammatory, like grains. We do not know the exact mechanism behind milk's apparent ability to trigger inflammation, but we do know that it is a metabolic modifier.

Milk is the food that provides for metabolic transition from being fed umbilically in the womb to the ability to eat whole foods or the kind of foods that the person is going to be able to eat for the rest of their life. Milk is not one of these foods—humans do not generally have affinity to drinking fresh milk on a long-term basis. Milk is filled with a number of metabolic modifiers which prompt babies to go through certain changes, like growing as fast as possible. This type of role is necessary in infancy, but once the infant has been weaned and has moved to whole food or regular food, milk becomes inappropriate. In fact, the high levels of proteins like insulin-like growth factor (IgF) found in dairy products can cause harm in our bodies once past weaning.

The body actually has a gene which generates milk intolerance.

The body actually has a gene which generates milk intolerance. The effect is to basically keep the child from returning to milk as a food supply. There are some areas of the world, like certain northern European and southern African locations, where their populations appear to be able to keep the milk intolerance gene from becoming active. The theory is that once agriculture and animal husbandry developed there, the climate was cool enough to store milk as a food supply. The generations that followed had a constant supply of milk, and so developed the genetics to keep that gene from shutting off the ability to digest milk as adults.

You will find, though, that people in almost any population who go off milk for a long enough period will develop intolerance to some degree. Again, this brings to mind the study about chronic earaches in small children where fresh milk was one of the sources thought to cause chronic inflammation.

Fortunately, many people can still enjoy dairy on BalancePoint if the dairy has been prepared correctly. We do not use fresh milk or direct fresh milk products, but do use strained "Greek-style" yogurt and low-fat feta cheese. After the two-week Jumpstart program we introduce hard, mature cheeses like true Parmagiana (not the processed grated version found in Parmesan shakers), which is a reduced fat cheese therefore lower in cholesterol and saturated fats. The problematic proteins which affect metabolism are soluble. So when you strain the yogurt, the whey drains out carrying these proteins away in the process. This whey, and therefore the metabolic modifiers, have already been drained out of hard cheeses.

Also, the fermentation process used to make the cheese probably breaks down some of these metabolic modifiers and lactose. This results in a better tolerance for milk products such as feta cheese, which we recommend in its low-fat version. However, for people who have had problems with cheese and yogurt in the past, we recommend steering clear of both of these until the first two weeks of the protocol are done, and then testing these foods cautiously when reintroducing them to your diet.

My blood test results at the finish of the 2-weeks were mind boggling. Cholesterol dropped from 238 to 148. Triglycerides dropped from 146to 49. "Bad" LDLs dropped from 154 to 69. "Good" HDLs went up from 55 to 70. Being on BalancePoint has convinced me that this way of eating is giving me an opportunity to live a longer, more active life.

Dale K., Age 56

CHAPTER 11

Three fronts for fighting cardiovascular disease

The BalancePoint protocol fights cardiovascular disease on three fronts:

(i) It reduces inflammation so that artery walls become less stiff, more flexible.

(ii) It lowers the amount of LDL cholesterol in the bloodstream.

(iii) It reduces inflammation so that the walls of the arteries are less vulnerable to invasion by damaging, small particle LDLs.

The BalancePoint protocol fights cardiovascular disease on three fronts

There are four mechanisms which BalancePoint uses to decrease the amount of cholesterol in our vascular system:

One, which we have discussed extensively, is the use of high fat levels to activate lipid metabolism and keep it continually running. The enzymatic pathways that metabolize or break down fat for energy also break down cholesterol.

The **second** is the employment of the high amounts of fat to prompt the body's preference for using cholesterol to make bile salts and sterols for digestion—a survival function—rather than LDLs for repair work—a lesser priority.

The **third** is the diet's minimal amounts of protein because periodic cutback of protein seems to cause scavenging of LDLs for recycling.

The **fourth** mechanism involves lowering inflammation, which, as we have explained in the last chapter, lowers the demand for LDLs to come in to do repair work

So more LDLs get used up in these four ways instead of floating around in the bloodstream. The problem with the LDL level in the arteries is seen in the amount of the small, dense particle LDLs, which are the ones depleted of their cholesterol load. These are the particular LDLs which are tiny enough to infiltrate into the arterial walls. Once inside, they can form lesions and plaque, the precursor of heart disease and strokes.

That is why BalancePoint's strong anti-inflammatory action is significant: It prevents and heals inflamed arterial walls so they are less easily penetrated by these particles.

The anti-inflammatory properties come from two mechanisms:

First, inflammatory triggers such pro-inflammatory foods like grains and fresh dairy are avoided.

Secondly, fats have recently been found to manufacture "resolvins" which both attenuate and terminate inflammation. Needless to say, the BalancePoint protocol is heavy in fat content.

The end result of BalancePoint's nutritional shift is not only dramatically improved numbers on the lipid panel—such as cholesterol, triglycerides, amount of small particle LDLs—at the doctor's office. By addressing the root of the problem, chronic inflammation, BalancePoint also produces better numbers for people on a whole series of cardiometabolic biomarkers, including abdominal obesity, elevated blood pressure, insulin resistance or glucose intolerance.

There is no doubt that the body is an amazing piece of evolutionary machinery, able to do incredible things **if used as designed**, in a way compatible with our ages-old genetic development.

And you can jumpstart your body into that mode!

BalancePoint–Harnessing the body's evolutionary wisdom

PART FOUR

Beating the hunger games

Why weight loss is easier through BalancePoint

The BalancePoint protocol allows for easy, significant weight loss, if losing weight is one of your goals.

Unlike traditional diets aimed primarily at weight reduction, the goal of BalancePoint is the rapid reduction of risk factors which are grouped together under the umbrella of cardiometabolic disease. So we see conditions such as high cholesterol and triglycerides, high blood glucose levels, high blood pressure, and stiff arteries improve dramatically in two weeks. In addition, however, many participants tell us that weight reduction is one of the more remarkable benefits of BalancePoint. In fact, many tell us that BalancePoint is the best program they have ever tried for shedding belly fat and excess pounds.

BalancePointers who want to lose weight typically lose five to fifteen pounds during the two-week Jumpstart program. Those who want to continue losing weight usually find themselves shedding an additional ten to twenty pounds over the next couple months as BalancePoint becomes a lifestyle.

By simply following the protocol, a BalancePointer's weight tends to naturally adjust to the right weight for him or her on its own. Some participants in the diet who prefer to gain pounds find that their weight gently rises to an appropriate level. The great thing about BalancePoint is that you have control over weight management so that ***you can tailor your***

program to lose, maintain or gain weight, and whichever way you go you still get the same amount of cardiometabolic improvement mentioned earlier.

Conventional diets, because of the biochemistry of their approach, produce cycles of starving between every meal and the suffering that goes along with them. It is hard to lose weight that way. BalancePoint offers a more comfortable solution, one that is less of a brute force and deprivation approach. This difference is due to three factors.

Adrienne H. has lost 150 pounds in three years on the BalancePoint Protocol. She says, "This is not a diet—it's my Live-it!"

She has incorporated the BalancePoint Wellness Lifestyle into not just her everyday living, but also her travels around the world. Wherever she goes, she manages to eat BalancePoint-style, even in countries where people cannot imagine a meal without rice or pasta.

At home, one of her favorite dishes is to steam asparagus and toss it with a dressing made of olive oil, lemon juice, crushed clove or two of garlic, salt, pepper, and a sprinkling—not too much because of the strong flavor—of chopped sundried tomatoes and Feta cheese. Makes a beautiful presentation for a reception or special dinner—along with Adrienne's new waistline and glow of health.

Flip the switch to burn fats instead of carbs

The first has to do with how BalancePoint encourages the body to burn fat instead of its preference to burn carbohydrates. Most weight loss diets are low-fat and high-carbohydrate diets. The primary source of calories is then carbohydrates. After each meal you either burn off the carbs you have just eaten, or convert them to store as fat so they can be later burned as a secondary source of calories.

The body gives priority to burning carbohydrates before fat. So when there are a lot of carbohydrates around to burn, the body is not motivated to switch from the carbohydrate metabolic pathway to the fat- or lipid-burning metabolic pathway. Since most overweight people are carbohydrate burners they do not have well-developed lipid-burning metabolisms. To be able to actually lose weight, you have to burn fat to burn off body fat.

As we have been pointing out, the secret to success of the BalancePoint protocol is keeping the body in lipid metabolism. You end up burning different types of lipids: the blood fat that is cholesterol and triglycerides, the fat in the belly area which is metabolically active and can produce hormones and chemical signals causing inflammation, and—most pertinent to this chapter—the fat that is being stored as a future energy source.

It is not just the fact that the body is switched to burning these stored fats that makes the pounds or waist inches go away more readily. There is also the issue of this continual lipid metabolism making it easier for people to keep on a diet, as I am about to explain.

Traditional diets set up starvation process—difficult to overcome

So what happens when you run out of carbohydrates to burn, like when you are on a low calorie or low fat diet? As I have just explained, the dietary source of calories, rather than the stored body fats, has to be used up first, with the carbohydrate metabolic pathway happily obliging. When the carbs run out there is an incredible craving for additional carbohydrates and a very strong drive to eat. It is the body's response to being starved. The lipid metabolism has to be started up to access the next source of calories. This switching over takes a period of time and the body goes through a pretty strong energy dip.

In a normal day for a person on a low-fat diet, he or she has to go through this excruciating transition after every meal: once the carbohydrates have been consumed the dieter gets that feeling of extreme, ravenous hunger, while insulin levels drop and the body slowly brings lipid or fat metabolism up to speed. No wonder the traditional dieting process becomes so difficult. You are continually going into starvation mode and your body is screaming at you to get another bagel at any cost! You have to go through this transition many times a day, which is quite uncomfortable and hard on a person's energy level.

These hunger rages and energy dips do not occur, though, when the body is already in the lipid metabolism, as when you are on BalancePoint. This is the second factor that makes BalancePoint an easier way to lose weight. You are in lipid metabolism already, and as you run through your dietary fat, you

---

BalancePoint is not a deprivation diet

have already started to mobilize and burn body fat supplying fuel to the metabolic pathway. It is a smoother and more even transition from using the dietary source of calories to the mobilization and utilization of body fat. Just as the shift is much less painful, the hunger is much less ravenous. The body does have the experience of hunger but it is much more subtle and it is not nearly the driving force as it is in a carbohydrate-burning mode.

The second important factor is that carbohydrates in the BalancePoint diet have a low-glycemic index. This means that they do not spike blood sugar levels which cause elevated insulin levels in the body. When insulin levels are high, the body cannot access fat in the cells to burn and so the fat stays stored there.

Dieting becomes a much easier process when the insulin levels are low. This way, the insulin is kept in a regulatory mode and not spiked into a mode of carbohydrate metabolism, which promotes storing of fat, instead of a lipid metabolism mode, which burns fat.

The swelling in my feet went down and my feet quit hurting. My joints don't hurt any more and that discovery was amazing for me. The 10 pounds I lost has stayed off effortlessly, and that's been huge. I wasn't thinking about food and wanting it. Never in my life have I just eaten and not worried about whether it'll make me gain weight. It's been liberating and I feel great.

SHERRY H., AGE 57

The third factor is that there are no grains in the diet. As we discussed in Chapter 10, grass-like grains such as wheat, oats, barley and rice contain a small protein called a lectin. This particular type of lectin is basically a poison pill, a defensive device to protect the plant from predators. Unfortunately, this protective mechanism also causes problems in many humans, probably about 80%, as far as we can tell in our research.

Lectins are very sticky and when they get into the bloodstream they attach themselves to receptor sites that act as monitors of insulin levels. As a result, the "gauges" get blocked and it takes a lot more insulin to get them to register the presence of insulin. In fact, by the time the receptors can sense the levels of insulin, the levels are inappropriately high. The body thinks there is less insulin than there really is and so keeps producing more.

Insulin is a very delicately balanced hormone, with extensive effects on the body's metabolic and vascular systems, so too high levels can be very problematic. In terms of this chapter on weight loss, our attention is drawn to the role of insulin to control the movement or mobilization of fat out of tissues such as the liver to be used as an energy source. If the body becomes insensitive to the levels of insulin, perhaps because lectins are interfering with the receptor sites, then it is not drawing out the fat for burning up.

Scientists also believe that the lectin proteins are sticking to the receptor sites for the hormone with a similar-sounding name, *leptin*. Leptin is one of the hormones that is used as a signal to tell us when we have had enough to eat. It is released as fat builds up in the body. When its levels reach a certain point, leptin says to the body, "We have enough food. We have enough stored to feel satisfied. We are not hungry."

In this way, our leptin sensitivity decreases so that we do not have the metabolic regulator to keep us within proper weight range.

When the insulin and leptin hormone system is knocked out or diminished in effectiveness, our natural regulatory systems get out of balance. We lose our sense of satiation that tells us we have had enough and the process of how and what foods are metabolized is disrupted.

We have huge amounts of refined grain products in virtually everything we eat in our modern Western diet, whether it is bread or pasta or thickeners in sauces. As a result, we are constantly exposed to high carbohydrate loading, which causes too rapid digestion and production of sugar in the body, and to the lectins in the grains. When you look at the biochemical effects, it is not too surprising then that we end up with chronic obesity in our society. The bad news is that it is an epidemic affecting our children.

The good news is we can do something about it. Are you ready to take that journey?

Dieting does not have to mean feeling hungry.

PART FIVE

The BalancePoint Protocol

What it is and how to follow it

Now we get to the heart of why you have picked up this book. You are no doubt wondering, what exactly is the BalancePoint dietary protocol? How do I use it to lose belly fat and pounds, or lower my LDL "bad" cholesterol by as much as 40 to 70 mg/dl, or get off my medication for arthritic pain, or normalize my blood glucose levels? How do I get back the elasticity of younger arteries? And see significant results in just two weeks?

The simple response is that BalancePoint is an anti-inflammatory diet which uses everyday foods in a very precise formula or protocol. By lowering inflammation in the body, this protocol gets to the source of many chronic conditions, as explained in previous chapters.

If you follow our protocol *as specified*, you will often begin seeing results in only a few days.

We call the initial two weeks of the Balance Point protocol our "Jumpstart" program.

It is easy to try. You can find whatever you need at the local supermarket. So here are a few general points about the BalancePoint protocol:

- It consists of common, everyday foods.
- It does not require esoteric nutrients or supplements, other than Omega 3 fish oil tablets and any kind of multivitamins.
- It does require your meals and snacks to fit into a precise nutritional formula; the 2-week Jumpstart program helps you develop this knowledge and skill.

- You can make the regimen ultra-simple with a routine of a few basic meals with easy variations. As one woman told us, it is appealing to have this I-do not-have-to-think-or-decide option, at least for the initial two-week Jumpstart.
- Or you can get creative and dress up meals into gourmet and multi-ethnic cuisine. (We have included recipes for both approaches.)
- Either way, your meals and snacks can fit the BalancePoint formula to give you great health results, and we will tell you how you can still follow it whether you are at the airport food court or at stopping at a roadside diner. The high fat content makes the meals tasty and satisfying, so that you do not feel the hunger or deprivation associated with conventional dieting.

And, even though BalancePoint is comprised of ordinary foods, we encourage you to consult your doctor or health practitioner before starting the protocol, and especially if you are on medications.

Since we are talking about food plans, it is important to make the distinction that BalancePoint is a protocol and not a diet in the sense of what "diet" means to most people, who tend to want to compare BalancePoint to other diets like South Beach or Atkins.

At age 64 I can hardly remember feeling or looking better. I've always looked quite a bit younger than my age but what I didn't feel was good energy. I had low blood sugar and often I would get shaky and feel kind of faint. I would grab a piece of cheese or some kind of protein to keep from feeling shaky and fainty.

Since I've been religious about BalancePoint I NEVER have those blood sugar spikes and even though I get a bit winded walking up a hill when I'm on the golf course, I never feel like my energy has been sapped.

BalancePoint has given me an entirely new way of eating. Dropped my cholesterol to 143. Dropped my weight from 126 to 116 and my energy is through the roof.

Jackie W.

CHAPTER 12

Why is BalancePoint a protocol and how is it different from a diet?

Protocol
prō'tō-kol:
A formula; a precise and detailed plan for a treatment regimen.

When most people think "diet" their interest is weight loss. Weight loss happens to be a happy by-product of our protocol and many people tell us it is the easiest way to lose weight they have ever found. But, if you do not want to lose weight, you do not have to. Some people actually are able to gain desired weight for the first time in their adult lives. It doesn't matter—whether you lose, maintain or gain weight you still get the same rapid cholesterol reduction. The point is that with the BalancePoint protocol, *you are in control.* You can usually have power over how much, if any, weight you lose, plus to some extent, how quickly.

For most people, losing weight is one of the secondary goals of going on our program, even if it is only five pounds. However, the focus of the BalancePoint protocol is more fundamental and comprehensive. It produces an ideal environment in the body to allow it to repair itself rapidly.

To accomplish this, the protocol is science-based. There is precision in the protocol related to layers of science. Each of the elements makes specific biochemical changes.

We get remarkable results from this precision. BalancePoint basically amounts to a formula or prescription of everyday foods. That is why it is critical to accurately monitor and track the amount and type of all the food you eat—down to the gram level—to make sure you are operating within this formula. The initial shift in metabolism requires two weeks of scrupulous attention, and, for some, an aggressive lifestyle change. So it is not for everyone.

But those who have carefully adhered to it have outstanding results. Many tell us that the biggest plus is finding a newfound feeling of empowerment. They have the experience of being able to control aspects of their health which they did not know they could have power over. These benefits are powerful enough to convince people to make eating Balance Point-style their new way of life.

And, by the way, after a couple weeks of the "pain-in-the-butt" careful measuring of your food and using an online tracking and calculating tool, you will develop an intuitive feel for portion size. Think of it as a two-week training process. You will then need to check yourself maybe only once or twice a month to keep up the skill. People have told us they can develop a sense for pouring out an amount of olive oil accurate to the gram!

BalancePoint:

A PRECISE FORMULA of managed calories, very high fat, minimum protein & low-glycemic carbohydrates

THE MOST IMPORTANT NOTE IN THIS BOOK!

BalancePoint is NOT a pick-and-choose approach!

Meticulous attention and compliance is the key to making the metabolic shift which gives BalancePoint its quick and remarkable results. But it is attention to, and compliance with, a food **formula**.

These are not general dietary guidelines for you to follow as you wish. They are part of ***a detailed and specific regimen which we know works—but in the way it has been set up. To obtain the results we talk about, you need to follow the protocol exactly as we have designed it***. We find that whenever people make changes, the results change—and not for the better. Reducing the amount of olive oil by only 1½ tablespoons a day can affect your results by as much as 50%. It is like altering a prescription.

You are either on the protocol or not. If you find yourself saying you are "half-way" or "mostly" on it, you are simply "not" on it. You may still get the kind of results which will please your doctor, reductions such as a 10 or 20 mg/dl in "bad" LDL cholesterol, which dwarf the numbers achieved by traditional diets. But people can usually get a 40 to 70 or higher mg/dl drop—***four times*** as much—on BalancePoint. To do so, they need to be completely on the protocol by measuring, logging and calculating all their food intake daily for the two week Jumpstart initiation.

As my mother-in-law likes to say,"No ifs, ands or buts!"

So it is important that you do not go into this chapter thinking that you can pull out a few main features of the protocol—the parts you like—and you will be on BalancePoint.

There is no getting around the measuring and logging to see where you stand and know if you are indeed following the protocol. In other words, within the ***numbers***, not just the kinds of foods.

For those of you who might have strong ideas about food and are tempted to alter the protocol, we encourage you to try the protocol exactly like it is for the two weeks. Then go ahead and experiment. It is easy to get a blood test to see if you get the same results. But until then, do it the way we know works!

CHAPTER 13

Overview of the BalancePoint Protocol

The BalancePoint protocol uses food to biochemically shift your metabolism and keep the fat—and cholesterol—burners going. To do this, BalancePoint uses a high-fat, minimum-protein, non-glycemic carbohydrate, and managed-calorie formula.

That will mean eating some types of food, like olive oil, in amounts you probably never imagined. Olive oil and other fats like nuts and avocados will become your new staple and primary source of calories instead of bread, pasta, rice or potatoes.

Yes, you read that right. There will be ***no*** grains—***no*** bread, ***no*** pasta, ***no*** rice.

If you read the previous chapters you will understand the reason for this prohibition. For some people, their first reaction is that this is a deal-breaker. But we continually hear that the thought of giving up grains is a lot more difficult than the act.

Chart 1. Quick Summary

BALANCEPOINT PROTOCOL

The metabolic pathway to health:
Fight fat with fat and extinguish inflammation

High fat, minimum protein, low-glycemic carbs
70% Fat, plus or minus 5%
40-50 grams Protein (~10% of calories)
20-25% Low-Glycemic Carbs
(greens, vegetables, some fruit)
NO Grains
NO Dairy (except strained yogurt and Feta)
Lots of spices for taste
Red wine, dark chocolate, coffee all OK
Managed Calories ±1200

+ Exercise
+ Reduce Stress

See also Chart 2: Two-week Jumpstart program and Chart 3: Wellness Lifestyle

On the other hand, the high fat content means you will not be dealing with hunger pangs common to most diets and nutritional programs. This is not a deprivation diet—and you will be able to create and eat a lot of delicious dishes. The fat will help keep you feeling full and can carry a lot of spices and flavorings in your dishes.

Many of you may already eat in a similar way. For others, it is a new experience in healthy eating. We joke about one of our early protocol

The BalancePoint Food Pyramid

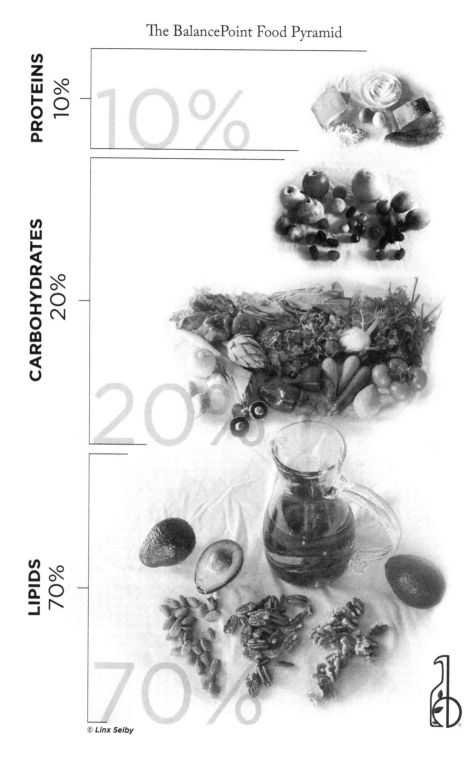

© Linx Selby

participants for whom "vegetables" meant "the green and red stuff you take off the hamburger before you eat it." (No, he did not immediately change his lifestyle to comply with BalancePoint guidelines, but he is inching closer and closer with a little change here, and another there...)

Even if you are already eating a lot of the foods on our protocol, such as lots of olive oil and green vegetables with no grains, please note that it is the amounts and proportions which make or break your success—this is a formula! We cannot say often enough that simply pouring olive oil on a plateful of greens is not "being on BalancePoint."

Following our protocol will also mean a strict regimen of carefully measuring all the food you eat, down to the level of each gram, for two weeks to make sure it fits within the BalancePoint formula.

Yes, embarking on this protocol is demanding and requires work. But remember, this first step is only two weeks—a small investment which will become second nature and lead you into a sustained program of lifelong wellness.

With all this in mind, let's now look at what makes up the protocol. Note that what follows is primarily geared toward our two-week Jumpstart rapid cholesterol reduction program to initiate you into the longer term BalancePoint Wellness Lifestyle.

1. Healthy fats become the new staple

The scientific word for fats is "lipids." Whether you call them fats or lipids, these wonderful foods will become the staple of your diet. Americans typically choose high-glycemic carbohydrates such as bread, pasta, rice and potatoes as the staple for providing calories. Prepare yourself for a change. *You will be using fats like nuts, avocados and lots of olive oil instead to provide calories. These* ***"healthy" fats will make up 70% of your caloric intake, plus or minus 5%.***

The high fat or lipid content calls on the body to continually burn instead of storing fat or cholesterol, which happens when you are in carbohydrate metabolism. (For more discussion on the science of lipid metabolism refer back to Chapter 6.) All the fat in the diet also leaves you feeling satisfied and full without hunger cravings.

The fats we use in the BalancePoint protocol are primarily monounsaturated from olive oil (make sure it is extra virgin), avocados, nuts such as almonds, walnuts and other tree nuts, but not peanuts (which are actually a legume rather than a nut), and certain seeds. We chose these because they are considered "healthy fats".

Olive oil (or canola oil until you develop an acceptance of, or even a preference for, olive oil) will be your primary source of lipids. Cook with it, slather it over everything—even fruit!—and *make sure you eat up all the oil that is left on your plate or in the pan because one tablespoon short will dramatically affect your total fat content.* You can see that for yourself by using an online nutritional tracker and calculator!

Try to take most of your olive oil portion in the morning, perhaps even half of the daily amount, to get your lipid metabolism going for the day.

We find it helpful to carry a little 75-100 gram bottle of olive oil with you so you can make sure you get your dose. Remember, do not assume that taking a certain amount of olive oil a day, such as 75 grams, puts you on the BalancePoint protocol. It is the calculation of its percentage of your total calories that counts, and the amount of olive oil will change depending on other lipids and foods you eat during the day.

2. No grains or grain products

This may be the most challenging aspect of the protocol for many people—no bread, pasta, cereals, wheat, oatmeal, barley, spelt, corn, or rice. We ask you to be vigilant in avoiding even tiny amounts of grains, such as sauces made with cornstarch or gravies made with flour.

We originally excluded these monocot or grass-like grains from the protocol because of their high glycemic index/load, which means they tend to raise glucose or blood sugars fast. By the way, did you know that bread breaks down immediately and raises blood sugar in your body? It breaks down faster than sugar, actually!

GLYCEMIC INDEX

The glycemic index rates how quickly a dietary carbohydrate turns into sugar in the blood stream, compared to a control food that's known to turn into blood sugar fast , such as white bread or pure glucose. For example, if 24 grams of pure glucose is rated at 100, and a raw apple containing 24 grams of carbohydrate has a glycemic index of 38, it means the blood glucose response to the carbohydrate in the apple is 38% of the blood glucose response to the same amount of carbohydrate in pure glucose. The fiber in an apple slows down sugar absorption, and that's why it has a lower glycemic index.

However, during our early research, we experimented with re-introducing low-glycemic grains that turn into sugars more slowly, such as steel-cut oats, whole grains and brown rice. After just one week of adding in these whole grains, we saw the levels of LDL "bad" cholesterol increasing by 50%. In other words, half of the cholesterol improvement achieved after the two-week BalancePoint Jumpstart program was lost by simply adding in these widely used starches.

In comparison, another group of participants were given small amounts of meat or fish to eat daily for a week, and their LDL levels increased only slightly.

GLYCEMIC LOAD

The glycemic load was developed to simultaneously describe the quality (glycemic index) and quantity of carbohydrate in a meal or diet. For instance, eating one apple gives you a relatively low glycemic load. Three apples at once would triple the load and be more likely to raise blood sugars.

For more information: Glycemic Index and Glycemic Load, by Jane Higdon, Ph.D., Linus Pauling Institute, Oregon State University

This is contrary to what I had expected. The meat and fish contain cholesterol, so I had thought that their effect on raising LDLs would be greater than that of grains, which contain no cholesterol. I concluded that there was a factor in grains and, as discussed in Part III, I believe it to be a little protein called a lectin.

The vast majority of cholesterol flowing through the bloodstream does NOT come from our diets. It is produced by your liver, then packaged into forms like LDLs, to help the body with maintenance, repair and energy utilization. The more inflammation in the body, the more need for repair. Because a primary purpose of cholesterol is to help with tissue repair, it may be that high LDL levels indicate an overload of inflammatory damage. When grains increase inflammatory damage, the body calls for repair crews of cholesterol to come in, thus raising LDL levels.

One of the more obvious signs of inflammation is arthritic pain. If you are starting to feel renewed arthritic pain which had previously gone away on the two-week protocol, you may be slipping in vigilance about avoiding grain or getting enough oil. Even the breading on onion rings or the tiny wheat content in soy sauce can trigger a noticeable inflammatory response in people who are especially sensitive to this inflammatory effect of grains. And if you are reading this book because of high cholesterol, belly fat or metabolic syndrome, there is a very good chance you are one of these people. You may not have known it before going on the protocol!

After your biomarkers have reached healthy levels on our two-week Jumpstart program, it is essential that you continue to avoid grains in your new BalancePoint Wellness Lifestyle. You might take a vacation from the protocol on special occasions and indulge in some grains. We can see on our arterial stiffness-measuring device that the age of your arteries can increase by thirty years or so within a day of eating grains. However, once you've reached a healthy baseline on BalancePoint, the recovery is much faster. If you return to the no-grains protocol, you will see your arterial age—and arthritic pain—reduce once more within days. So after the rigorous two-week Jumpstart, if you take a protocol vacation for a special event, go back completely, not just "mostly," to avoiding all grains. Whatever you do, **never combine high glycemic foods with fats**. Do not think you are staying on the protocol by pouring olive oil on your bread or potatoes. That is a deadly combination and if you are going to eat high-glycemic foods go to a low-fat diet. Otherwise, your insulin levels will be driven up, your body will try to store rather than metabolize fat, and weight gain will result.

Whatever you do, never combine high glycemic foods with fats. Do not think you are staying on the protocol by pouring olive oil on your bread or potatoes.

In the words of someone who has lost 150+ pounds and arthritic pain on the BalancePoint protocol, it is difficult to explain to people how going grain-less is truly possible. They have to try it themselves. We get surprised comments all the time from former bread- or bagel-addicts who find that, once they got through the first few days, it becomes easier than they ever imagined to go cold-turkey. You might be one of them! You might in fact become one of the people who tell us things like, "When I taste a cookie now all I can taste is the flour and sugar," or "When I had a piece of bread I could actually feel it heavy in my stomach."

It goes without saying that *you are not home free if you simply reach for gluten-free products.* These foods are usually made with rice or oats or corn, also to be avoided on the BalancePoint protocol. Restaurants have become much more gluten-free conscious in the past few years, and often mark their menus accordingly. That gets you part of the way, but *you still need to ask about the other grains and rice or corn starches, which are often used for coating or thickening.*

In fact, you will become, perhaps for the first time in your life, a label-reader. It is eye-opening to see how often you find flour and cornstarch on the list of ingredients. As mentioned, they are used as a coating for or thickener in many foods, often when you least suspect it. Common culprits are salad dressings, soups, regular not strained yogurt, soy sauce, and even sweet potato fries which are usually coated.

3. Minimum, not excessive protein

We restrict the amount of protein to the minimum needed for bodily maintenance and repair. These levels keep the protein from being used as a calorie source and thus being broken down into sugars and nitrogenous waste, which the body cannot use.

Our protocol calls for 40 (plus or minus 5) grams protein, which usually works out to less than 10% of your daily calories (closer to 15% if you are at the 1200 calorie level). We have found that restricting the protein leads to larger drops in LDL "bad" cholesterol.

We discovered this phenomenon of **minimum protein=lower LDLs** when one of our first participants reduced her LDLs by a mind-boggling 70 mg/dl points after 14 days on BalancePoint. When we looked at her food logs, we saw that she was inadvertently eating less protein than what we were recommending at that time. So we have found over the past almost six years that when someone needs very aggressive LDL drops, keeping the protein at the lower end, from 35-40 grams/day is a good strategy.

To minimize saturated fats and cholesterol during the two-week Jumpstart of the Protocol, we specify no meat or fish as protein sources during this period only. The exception is one small serving (55 grams or 2 ounces) of salmon somewhere around Day 7 to add some variety to the diet—a treat,

> *"BalancePoint is not a diet—it's a live-it"*
>
> - Adrienne H. (has lost 150 lb, still losing)

if you will. Remember, only on Day 7 of the 14 days, and not on any of the other days. On other days, most of your protein will come from cholesterol-free sources such as egg whites, which are considered the perfect protein (ideally balanced in amino acids because they are designed to support the development of an embryo), tofu, strained yogurt, or tiny amounts of feta cheese. Nuts, almond butter, and even the cocoa and some vegetables also contribute protein and may play a factor in your overall protein totals.

When new Jumpstart dieters tell us they are feeling weak, agitated, dizzy, or "spacey", and having trouble sleeping, we often find that they are not reaching their minimum 35 or 40 grams of protein per day.

After the two-week Jumpstart program, when you are on the BalancePoint Wellness Lifestyle, you will be able to add other sources of protein, such as *fish, grass-fed buffalo or grass-fed beef (see Chapter 16). But you must remember to keep under 45 total grams of protein per day, even if you have raised your calorie levels, which, if you do raise, you should do only slightly.*

4. Avoiding cholesterol in food

Greens, greens, and more greens!

Our protocol eliminates almost all sources of external cholesterol in the two-week Jumpstart portion of the program. This optimizes cholesterol reduction, leaving the body to function primarily on the cholesterol it produces itself. Not adding dietary cholesterol cuts down the load of cholesterol that needs to be metabolized or eliminated to achieve reduction within the body. So we exclude animal products as sources of dietary cholesterol. After the initial two-week period with cholesterol numbers now in balance, these protein sources are added back into the diet in moderation and keeping to the same ratio of protein percentage of total calories, as described above.

Egg yolks, another source of dietary cholesterol, are also eliminated in the Jumpstart two weeks for the same reason. *For those people whose cholesterol levels are at a desired level and do not need to get their cholesterol numbers down, egg yolks can be added after this period in moderation, such as once or twice a week.* In this case, it is a good idea not to break or scramble the egg yolks when cooking because that action allows the LDLs to oxidize. This makes the LDLs more problematic in the arteries and increases arthrogenesis.

5. How do we get enough carbohydrates?

While you will get most of your calories from fats instead of grains, you will still eat plenty of carbohydrates. Up to 20 to 25% of your calories (up to 80 grams) in fact will still be carbohydrates. However, they will be different than what most Americans are used to. Instead of sweet or starchy carbs such as soda and chips, or muffins and potatoes, you will be eating high-fiber carbs that are filled with healthy nutrients and which cause fewer sugar spikes in your bloodstream. Carbohydrates that quickly raise sugar levels in the bloodstream are called "high glycemic" (the word glycemic come from glucose, a form of sugar).

So on BalancePoint, you will not eat high glycemic foods (see below.) Instead, you will reach for the *low-glycemic carbs... high fiber vegetables that are delicious with generous splashes of olive oil, such as salad greens, eggplant, kale, mushrooms and red peppers, plus low glycemic fruits such as apples, pears and berries.* Because so many of these are low in calories, you can have heaping plates of salad and generous portions of eggplant and mushrooms sautéed with olive oil and garlic, which are delicious meals.

Huge salads are in fact what we recommend for your daily lunch or dinner meal. Adding lots of olive oil makes the salad far more filling. You can get creative adding greens such as spinach or fennel—or leftovers from last night's stir-fry! Or add vegetables such as poblano chilies and peppers plus some nuts to make a more substantial salad.

6. Plant-based nutrients

Fruits, nuts and vegetables have been in our diet as it has evolved over millions of years. They contain a large variety of phytonutrients, which confer many protective—one could say almost magical—qualities for the benefit of our health. There are many medical studies of the effect of phytonutrients on reducing the risk of chronic disease, including coronary heart disease, stroke and cancer. As an example of their protective nature, the antioxidants found in the leafy greens and the skins of berries help defend the plant against solar damage and then in turn guard us from oxidative and free radical damage to our cells.

So, "An apple a day" and Grandma's admonishing to eat all your green vegetables still stands as valuable advice. Our protocol incorporates lots of phytonutrient-rich foods like green salads, dark leafy green vegetables, such as kale, chard, turnip greens, and bok choy, and certain fruit, especially apples and berries. *Adding greens to egg whites in the morning is a great way to get green vegetables into your meal plan as early as possible in the day.*

7. No high-glycemic foods

Foods such as grains, potatoes, carrots, watermelon and bananas cause a rapid rise in blood sugar. This causes a spike in levels of a hormone called insulin. High insulin levels signal the body to convert carbohydrates that are not burned for energy into fat (triglyceride) for storage, predominantly in your middle—the pot belly we all know of. *The insulin spike also stops the lipid metabolism we are trying to maintain and turns your lipid burner down and sometimes even off. What is more, frequent insulin spikes promote inflammation in the body. So there are many reasons to reduce your glycemic load.*

I went on BalancePoint because I had open heart surgery ten years ago but my cholesterol was high. It took a couple tries to get into the BalancePoint mode but once my wife and I got into the protocol, it was surprisingly easy. And that's coming from someone who used to be on a potato chips, ice cream and beer diet. My doctors tell me now that my heart health is great. The added bonus is that whatever else was wrong is also getting fixed, such as PSA levels going way down.

JIM M., AGE 70

"Extra protein just turns into sugar and nitrogen compounds."

Because beans, such as lentils, garbanzo and pinto, and legumes, such as peanuts (!) and peas, often have a somewhat high glycemic load, they are not allowed during the two-week Jumpstart portion of the BalancePoint protocol. The only exception are fermented beans that are lower in carbs, such as tofu. Also, for another reason, there are some people who discover that legumes are pro-inflammatory for them. So we *eliminate beans, peanuts and peas during the two-week Jumpstart program.* For this first period we are trying to remove as many potential inflammatory triggers as possible. Most people will find they can add legumes after this period with no ill effects, unlike grains, which permanently stay on the no-fly list!

You may not be aware that juice, due to its concentrated sugar content, also falls into the high-glycemic category. Anyone who has made fresh-squeezed orange juice knows that it takes four oranges to make almost a cup of juice. So you are getting the concentration of the sugar of all those pieces of fruit. You might have seen recent headlines warning parents that fruit juice is ounce per ounce often more sugar-laden than sodas. *Avoid both fruit juice and dried fruit for this reason.* However, many low glycemic fruits eaten raw and whole are fine on the BalancePoint protocol because their mass of fiber slows down absorption of the sugar.

Sugars and sweeteners are obviously not allowed, except in extremely limited amounts, such as ¼ teaspoon in your cocoa drink. Many people ask about agave but it too is a fructose and, until further research indicates, should be avoided. This also means no salad dressings or sauces with sugar in them, and *no balsamic vinegar* for the same reason.

If you are worried about satisfying your sweet tooth, you may be in for a welcome surprise. After a few days of adapting to the BalancePoint diet, many participants report MORE flavor in their food. As taste buds adapt, foods that previously tasted bland now burst with more sweet notes, spiciness and pleasure.

To keep your fat-burners going strong, even these low glycemic carbohydrates will be no more than 20-25% of your daily calories. That is basically the balance of whatever is left after your 70% fat and 40-50 grams of protein.

8. Strained yogurt and feta rather than milk, fresh cheeses and regular yogurt

Most people do not realize that fresh milk can raise insulin levels, turn down your fat burners and promote inflammation. But it can, in a variety of ways.

Milk is called a low glycemic food, which generally does not lead to sugar spikes. However, it leads to insulin spikes, which increase insulin resistance and inflammation, the same way white bread does. White bread does it through sugar levels, milk does it directly.

What is more, milk and other dairy products carry metabolic modifiers which play a role in helping babies grow rapidly, but can cause an inflammatory reaction when we consume them past weaning.

Instead of fresh milk and cheeses, the BalancePoint protocol calls for ***strained*** *low-fat or non-fat yogurt and tiny amounts of low-fat feta cheese.* Note that we are beginning to see a lot more yogurt labeled "Greek-style", but not all "Greek style" is strained and some contain cornstarch, which is a grain product and therefore not allowed on the BalancePoint protocol. Straining away the liquid whey seems to remove the harmful metabolic modifiers which are pro-inflammatory, as explained in Chapter 10. So look for the word "strained" on the container. Do not get misled by thick-looking yogurts, such as Balkan style, without calling the 800-number on the label to confirm that they are strained. In our experience they usually are not.

You can buy the yogurt already strained in brands such as Fage, Oikos, Voskos, and Trader Joe's Greek Style. These brands are beginning to penetrate the market now and we have seen them at Costco (which has its own delicious Kirkland brand Greek yogurt), Safeway and even Walmart. Or do it yourself by letting a good quality yogurt such as Nancy's sit overnight in a coffee strainer and then disposing the liquid. You are left with a thicker, tarter, richer tasting yogurt.

> *"Fat calories do not count the same way as carb calories."*

Products made from whey, such as processed cheese should be avoided. This includes cottage cheese and all soft cheeses, even if they are low-fat. *For anyone wanting a milk-like drink, we suggest unsweetened almond milk.*

9. Calories and weight management

In recent animal research, the restricted caloric diet approach is being heralded for promoting longevity. Most people find such low-calorie diets too severe—it is difficult to keep starving. *The difference with the BalancePoint protocol is that, while it does restrict caloric intake, it is made up of a high fat content. This leaves you feeling full and satisfied, and makes our foods delicious and appealing.* We had to smile when one woman asked us, "I don't think I can get **up** to 1200 calories a day—I get such a satisfied feeling after eating the olive oil, avocados and nuts!"

Some recent research has indicated that it may not be so much the total calories but the type of calories which should be restricted, such as carbohydrates and protein. Fat calories do not count the same way as carb calories. So when looking at intake, BalancePoint calories may total higher than typical caloric-restricted diets but are in fact equivalent. It is important, nevertheless, to eat only the minimum calories needed to maintain healthy bodies.

The BalancePoint protocol begins by *kicking your metabolism into fat-burning mode at a level of 1200 calories a day for at least two days. This is to put some stress on the metabolic system to move it into gear more rapidly for the metabolic shifts BalancePoint is producing.* Even if your body is feeling some hunger—different than the typical diet starvation kind described earlier—during these couple days of transition it is good for the body to feel this type of tension as it re-adjusts to a different metabolism.

The protocol does a remarkably good job of managing your weight as well. Once you are in a lipid metabolism mode, that is, compliant with the protocol, you can easily manage the calories you eat each day by adjusting the amount of olive oil you consume or else by reducing your snacks. See Part IV, "Why Weight Loss is Easier on BalancePoint."

People who want to lose weight usually stay at this 1200 calorie level. If you are one of the few of want to maintain or gain weight, or if you are very active physically and you want to slow your rate of weight loss to a more gradual level, choose a target of 1300-1500 calories per day. In this case, increase your calorie level gradually, about 100 calories per day from the initial 1200 level, and watch to see whether you are still losing or maintaining pounds. This 1200 number is for a "typical" person and your base level may be different and need adjusting, depending on factors such as your level of physical activity. This is about finding your balance point, right?

In fact, when we monitor people on the two-week Jumpstart program we look at daily weight measurements as one indicator of how well someone is following the protocol. Everyone, regardless of whether they want to eventually lose or even gain weight, should drop a couple pounds in the beginning because the body is losing glycogen. Then people who want to shed some pounds—which is almost everyone—should show a half pound or one pound loss every one or two days.

Some people might even need to go below 1200 calories, down to 1000 or even 900, to reduce weight. This tends to be more an issue with women. But, whether men or women, they should monitor carefully what level keeps them losing weight every day and see how they feel.

People on BalancePoint who wish to lose weight often shed ten to fifteen pounds in the first two weeks. This is particularly true for men. And the even better news is that this reduction is seen in abdominal fat!

Belly fat is the most dangerous type of fat on the body because of its proximity to major organs like the liver. Almost everyone knows that it is extremely difficult to get rid of belly fat, no matter how much exercise or traditional starvation dieting. Now you have a solution: *BalancePoint targets belly fat* and you can often see a difference already in two weeks. In fact, if we see someone starting to get belly fat again we know he is off the protocol—a good clue!

The idea of 1200, or even less, calories may seem low, but this is another of those surprises which come after shunning grains. We invariably find people telling us that they were amazed to see, after the first two or three days, how they adjusted and realized they did not need more. They were just used to eating much more than they needed.

After the two week Jumpstart, increase your calories only after you reach your target weight and want to stop losing any more pounds.

Nonetheless, we recommend remaining attentive to your portion sizes, because people often report that they can eat less and have more energy, after the first two weeks on BalancePoint. ***While most people can eat a few hundred calories more than they need and still see their weight stay fairly stable, the improvements you have just achieved in your health do not stay at the same level.*** The body seems to work the best when it is fed on the lean side and you keep your caloric intake down at the bottom range of what you need.

"A diet that includes wine and dark chocolate? How can you not do it?!"

10. Red Wine, Tea, Coffee... and Chocolate!

If you wish, you can drink wine, tea and coffee, preferably red wine (no more than one to two glasses a day) and decaffeinated coffee. They actually contain some beneficial phytochemicals, such as the resveratrol found in red wine.

Because dark chocolate is high in flavanols and has some power to raise "good" HDL cholesterol, we recommend it on the BalancePoint protocol. As many people say, "A diet that includes wine and dark chocolate? How can you not do it?!" **But keep in mind that it is a very specific kind—unsweetened, non-alkalized cocoa** for its high content of a flavanol which improves blood flow in the cardiovascular system.

The "Dutch process" used for making milk chocolate does not retain the flavanols, so that is why

COCOA DRINK

15 g (2 heaping tablespoons) natural, non-alkalized (non-Dutch process), unsweetened cocoa powder
120-180 g unsweetened almond milk (make sure no rice starch in ingredients)

Heat the almond milk, add the cocoa and mix. An electric frother works great. Use the lesser amount of almond milk (or even less!) to make a thicker pudding-like treat. If you need to, use a tiny amount, no more than ¼ -½ tsp) of sugar, honey, agave or vanilla extract, when first getting used to the bitterness of the cocoa and then wean yourself off the sweetener (yes, it is possible!) 1 serving.

you need to be vigilant about the type of cocoa you use. Adding dairy milk to cocoa has the same effect and that is why we recommend almond milk instead. Some of the easiest types of this cocoa to find are Hershey's Natural Baking Cocoa or similar non-sweetened, non-alkalized cocoa made by other brands such as Ghiradelli. We recommend mixing our specified amounts of cocoa into a little bit of almond milk in a thick pudding-like mixture for a snack. However, if you are caffeine-sensitive, be aware that chocolate contains a caffeine-like stimulant so if it keeps you up at night, be sure to have your chocolate long before you head to bed.

One woman on BalancePoint said she gagged the first time she tried the non-sweetened drink and then got to a point where she craved it. Believe it or not, some people even like to add a little olive oil to the mixture. Yes, you will not only develop a taste for olive oil through all this. You may find yourself adding it in unforeseen ways to all kinds of foods.

After the two-week Jumpstart, you can start using dark chocolate with a 75-80% minimum of cacao content instead of the cocoa drink. By this time, though, you might find you too are looking forward to the cocoa drink.

11. Fiber and Fish Oil

The BalancePoint protocol is comprised of a great deal of vegetable fiber, both soluble and insoluble, which comes from vegetables and fruit. We add more fiber with psyllium fiber supplements in the morning and before bed. This fiber helps to carry away any unused cholesterol (more cholesterol is used for fat transport than is used for cell repair), so it will not be reabsorbed into the lower intestine. It is also beneficial if you are prone to constipation. You can find it in food stores, especially natural food stores. Take one heaping teaspoon twice a day, mixed in a little water or almond milk.

Two capsules of fish oil a day are suggested in this protocol, or you can get fish oil in liquid form and take a spoonful or two a day. Make sure you find a brand that has low cholesterol and is mercury free, has been molecularly distilled, and has a combined EPA and DHA (Omega3s) dosage of about 1.5 grams.

12. Exercise and Stress Reduction

The BalancePoint Wellness Lifestyle is made up of three cornerstones: nutrition, exercise and stress management. As you focus on nutrition, remember that exercise also plays a major role in maintaining physical and mental health and energy. Stress management can range from spiritual or meditative practices to enjoying time with friends and family, and is as vital as the other two parts of the triangle!

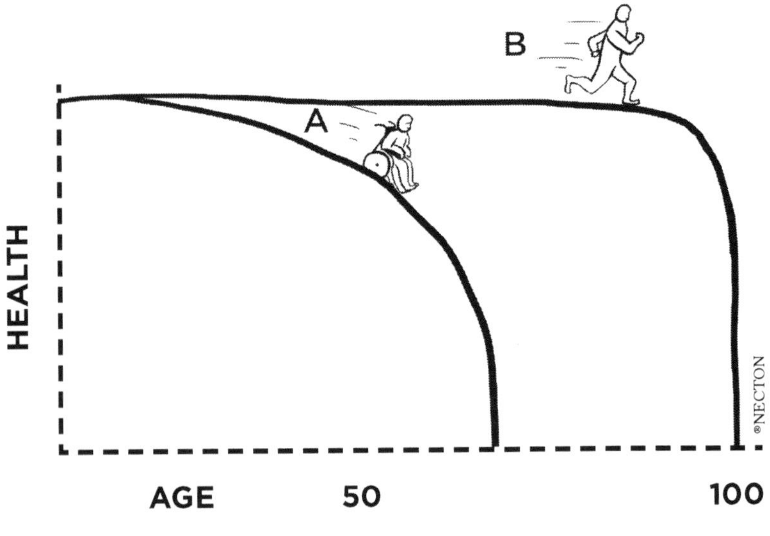

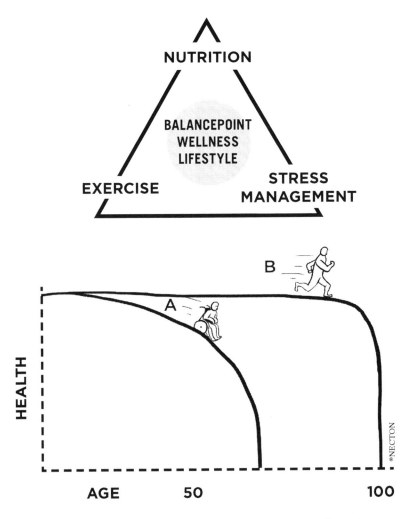

Health and Longevity can go hand-in-hand: as shown in this chart, the BalancePoint goal is robust longevity!

RECOMMENDED FOOD LIST

The BalancePoint Recommended Food List

VEGETABLE (Fresh or Cooked) *Lots of greens!*

Artichokes
Arugula
Asparagus
Avocado
Beet greens
Beets *(in limited quantity)*
Broccoli
Brussels Sprouts
Cabbage
Cauliflower
Celery
Chard
Chilies (*Fresh and Dried)*
Chinese *(Bok Choy)*
Collard Greens
Cucumber
Dandelion
Eggplant
Fennel Bulb
Fresh Herbs
Garlic
Ginger
Green Summer Squash
Greens
Kale
Kohlrabi
Mushrooms
Mustard Greens
Okra
Onions
Pepper (Bell)
Pepper Hot Chili
Poblano Pepper
Purslane
Radishes
Red Cabbage
Rutabaga
Seaweed
Spinach
Squash *(Yellow Summer)*
Sweet Potato *(Sautéed in limited quantity)*
Tomatoes
Turnip Greens
Turnips
Watercress
Zucchini

FRESH FRUITS *SMALL AMOUNTS. See Chart 2. Summary of the 2-week Jumpstart program*

Apple
Apricot
Blackberries
Blueberries
Boysenberries
Carambola
Cherimoya
Cherries
Clementines
Cranberries
Figs
Gooseberries
Grapefruit
Grapes
Guava
Kiwi
Lychee
Nectarine
Orange
Passion Fruit
Pears
Persimmon
Plums
Pomegranate
Raspberries
Rhubarb
Star Fruit
Strawberries
Tangerines
Tomatoes

OTHER FOODS

See Chapter 16 for foods allowed after 2 week jumpstart

Almond Milk - Unsweetened *(Blue Diamond)*
Almonds *(Raw and Unsalted Dry Roasted)*
Cocoa Powder – Non-Alkalized *(Hershey's Natural)*
Coffee and Espresso
Egg Whites
Eggplant *(Dip with Olive Oil)*
Green Tomato Chili Sauce *(Salsa Verde)*
Guacamole
Olive Oil
Salmon *(One time 4oz. serving on day 7 of 2 Week Jumpstart)*
Salsa
Tofu
Tomatoes *(Sun-Dried in Oil)*
Walnuts
Wine *(Dry Table)*
Yogurt - Strained Nonfat *(Fage 0%, Oikos, or Voskos)*

SEASONINGS

Herbs, spices, garlic, ginger, lemon and lime juice, etc. can be used in unlimited quantities, and do not need to be recorded on your food sheets.

NOT ON THE BALANCEPOINT PROTOCOL

Grains and Wholegrain

- Bread
- Pasta
- Cereals
- Oats
- Barley
- Millet
- Corn
- Flour
- Rice

Starches and Thickeners

- Cornstarch
- Flour Thickener
- Potato starch
- Thickened Dressings
- Thickened Soups

Cholesterol containing food

- Egg yolk
- Meat, fish, poultry

Not during 2 week Jumpstart, but allowed as per Chapter 16 after.

High Glycemic

- Balsamic Vinegar
- Bananas and watermelon
- Beets
- Carrots
- Fruit Juice
- Potatoes
- Sugars
- Sweetened Drinks
- Sweeteners

Dairy

- Butter
- Cheese*
- Cottage Cheese
- Milk
- Sour cream
- Yogurt**

Legumes

- Beans
- Lentils
- Peas
- Peanuts

Not during 2 week Jumpstart, but can add small amounts after if no adverse effects

** Except for low-cholesterol feta (e.g. Organic Valley brand)*
*** Except for strained non-fat yogurt such as Fage, Oikos, or Vosko*

CHAPTER 14

Doing the Protocol

Basic Supplies

- Gram Scale (available in many kitchen stores, or department stores like Target)
- Digital Body Weight scale with 1/10 pound measurements (The small increments are useful because, as explained earlier, a .5-pound of weight loss over a day is a good indication of how well you are complying with the protocol)
- Blood Pressure Cuff (It is a good idea to monitor your blood pressure while on the protocol. If you are taking high blood pressure medication to be sure to measure your blood pressure first thing in the morning and a couple of other times during the day, preferably once after some exercise. If BalancePoint lowers your blood pressure quickly you may need to consult with your doctor about reducing the dose of your medication.)
- Olive Oil Container (~90 grams for the whole day, or ~30 grams for a typical one-meal serving. Little camping bottles from an outdoors supply store work well.)
- Food Logging Chart (Do a daily log of your weight in 0.1 pounds, your blood pressure, and chart listing each food you eat or drink: Time, Quantity (in grams), and Name. Use this log as a basis several times a day to calculate the "How Am I Doing" chart on page 123.)

Pre and Post-Jumpstart Blood Tests to see what kind of results you get from the 2-week program

- **Cholesterol Test** - Get a prescription for what is called a Lipid Panel from your healthcare practitioner or contact a lab such as LabCorp or Quest directly to get a test without a prescription.
- We also highly recommend you include two other pre and post 2-week tests: **blood glucose and A1C**

- And because the actual size of LDL particles is a more accurate risk indicator than simply the level of LDL, the more sophisticated and detailed VAP or LipoScience NMR cholesterol tests are especially useful for those at high risk for cardiovascular disease.
- Changes on the BalancePoint protocol can happen very fast, so please **do not start changing your diet before going in for your first blood test.** Otherwise you will not have a true baseline to compare with.

IMPORTANT: The BalancePoint program is not intended to take the place of medical advice, so we recommend that you consult with your primary care health practitioner before starting our program. ESPECIALLY IF YOU ARE ON MEDICATIONS, consult with your physician. Some

Chart 2. Summary of the 2-week Jumpstart program

2-WEEK JUMPSTART PROGRAM

Summary of the 2-week Jumpstart program to quickly reduce cholesterol and inflammation

Patent pending. V.4.1, 2011-5-5

Remember that BalancePoint is a protocol, with a specific biochemical formula of macronutrients and a synergistic effect between all of its elements. You cannot pick and choose among the parts you like best. It is vital to precisely keep within the formula to achieve BalancePoint's spectacular results. To do this, use BalancePoint's or another online Nutrition/Wellness Tracker to make sure you are following the Protocol properly and accurately. It is the only way to know if you need an extra tablespoon of olive oil to get you from too-low 60% to just-right 70% fat, or if that apple is going to put you over the top in calories or carbs. There is no "sort-of" or "half-way." You are either within the formula or not. Being "80% compliant" will not get you 80% results; certain tipping points need to be reached for BalancePoint to work.

Fat = 70% of total calories *(min. 65%)*

Olive or canola oil, tree nuts, avocado, almond butter

40 grams Protein *(min. 35g, max. 45g)*

Egg whites, tofu, strained yogurt, feta cheese in very small quantities (10-15 g) used for seasoning only, nuts, greens, one-time small serving of salmon mid-program

Chart 2. Continued

Remaining calories after reaching above fat and protein targets come from
Low Glycemic Carbohydrates *(non-starchy and non-sugar)*
(less than 80 grams/day, no more than 20-25% of total calories)
Every meal, including breakfast, should generally include uncooked weight of 150 g (min. 125 g) of a salad or greens (important to use VARIETY for different nutrients), or tomatoes and non-starchy vegetables
Handful of berries (50-60 g) and most fruit, but in small quantity, e.g. one small apple
NO fruit juice, potatoes, bananas, watermelon, carrots

NO Grains
No wheat, oats, rice, corn, barley, millet, rice starch, cornstarch—check ingredients of soups, sauces and salad dressings [Note: "gluten-free" is usually not grain-free]

NO Legumes, *including peanuts, beans, peas*

NO Dairy *except strained yogurt and, for seasoning only, very small quantities of Feta cheese*
Almond milk or small quantities of soy milk OK

Lots of spices for taste
Red wine, coffee, tea all OK (no beer)
Cocoa (non-alkalized, non-sweetened) (Baking cocoa)
Fish oil and psyllium 2Xday, multi-vitamin

Restrict and manage calories
1200 first two days then adjust +/-100 calories/day if necessary, according to weight goals

+ Exercise
+ Reduce Stress

of the health changes on BalancePoint can occur so rapidly that it can be important to adjust medication doses. For instance, some participants on blood pressure medications report that their blood pressure drops low enough to reduce or eliminate that medication. The same often happens with people using medications for diabetes. And so on. So consult with your doctor.

Doing the Protocol

1. Measure

Measure everything in grams because you need the accuracy. Also, using a less familar unit of measure makes you more conscious of your measurements and not so likely to guess, as you might with "tablespoon" or "half a cup."

- Pre-breakfast and bedtime: 1 heaping teaspoon of **Psyllium**
- Pre-breakfast and bedtime: 15 grams unsweetened, non-alkalized **cocoa powder** in 120 grams almond milk
- With a meal: 2 **fish oil** Omega-3 pills
- **3 meals a day totaling ~1200 calories** (i.e. 350-450 calories per meal) **for days 1 and 2, then monitor your weight to decide whether to maintain or adjust 100 calories/day to 1500 calories thereafter. Whatever the calorie level, at the end of the day they must be composed of 70±5% fat and should also include 40±5 grams of protein.**

Tip: You can divide the calories evenly between your three meals, but most people find it helpful to make breakfast higher in both oil (40%-50% instead of one-third of your daily oil target) and protein (40% of daily protein target).

Breakfast - All breakfasts have a portion of oil (40-50% of your daily oil target if you are following above tip) to kick start lipid metabolism for the day and a portion of protein (40% of your daily total) to stabilize blood sugar.

Quick and Easy way to do it: Use > 30 g. olive oil in this meal and use it to cook two to three egg whites with 150 g. of vegetables, such as spinach or fresh tomatoes. Instead of bacon and eggs every morning, you can have egg whites and tomatoes with green onions—a simple breakfast solution for the two weeks.

Lunch and dinner - These meals are interchangeable and should be thought of as one meal with protein from sources like tofu, strained yogurt or egg whites (40% of your daily protein target) and one without protein (20% of your daily protein target coming from sources like nuts, almond butter, greens).

Both these meals should have large amounts of vegetables, such as salad, or cooked vegetables which you can serve on a bed of greens, such as romaine

HOW AM I DOING TODAY? *Fill in your numbers!*

	PROTEIN		FATS		CARBOHYDRATES		TOTAL CALORIES
	% cal.	g	% cal.	g	% cal.	g	
GOALS		*35-40 grams*	*>65-70 %*		*<25%*		*1200*
ACTUAL							

lettuce, if you like. Think of using greens rather than rice or pasta as a base for your dishes, and use dips like guacamole and strained yogurt for fresh vegetables like asparagus or endive.

Total protein for the day should be around 40 grams to ensure you are getting an adequate amount.

Quick and Easy way to do it:

i. Each of these meals should contain about 150-175 grams of non-starchy vegetables and the all-important 20 - 35 grams of olive oil (remember, for each meal, and make sure all oil from pan or dish is eaten).

ii. Prepare a salad for lunch everyday and sauté vegetables with tofu for every dinner. This is the simplest approach for the two-week program.

iii. Or use our pre-calculated recipes in Chapter 17.

Snacks - Use snacks to either increase or decrease your calorie levels. Note that at the 1200 calories/day level you may not be able to include the whole or any portion of snack because it could tip you over your calorie count. If you are at your weight goal and want to start increasing your calories, an easy way to do it is by adding one snack.

Quick and easy way to do it: Choose one of the following for one of the snacks. However, as per note above, you might have to decrease this by one-half or one-quarter:

- Half a fresh peach or 1 small apple with 7 grams of almond butter *Protein 1.3 g Fat 4.3 g, Carbs 16.1g. Calories 99.4*
- 25 grams of walnuts *Protein 3.8 g Fat 16.3 g, Carbs 3.4 g, Calories 163.5*

If you use the fruit or nuts in your salad meal, do not add more to your daily intake as a snack.

Some people make the mistake of thinking this is a protocol of taking a set amount, for example 75 or 100 grams, of olive oil a day. That is not true. *The amount will vary according to your end of the day tallies because of additional fat content you are getting from sources such like avocados or nuts, and because of your caloric level. That's why it's crucial to log and calculate since* **the important amount is 70% (+/- 5%), not a magic number of grams.**

2. Log and Calculate

Track all your food during the day and calculate the calories and lipid, protein and carbohydrate percentages at least twice a day to know where you stand so you can make appropriate adjustments and at the end of the day to make sure you are within the formula.

Quick and Easy way to do it:

i. Use a website tool to log and calculate how you are reaching your nutrient and calorie goals. You can go to the Lifestyle for Health Research Institute website www.LHRI.org to check availability of the online Nutrition/Wellness tracker and calculator shown in the "How Am I Doing Today?" chart on the previous page. It automatically calculates for you how much that serving of avocado or nuts or almond milk changes your extremely important lipid, protein and carbohydrate percentages of total calories. It gives you an instant running total you can check as often as you wish during the day. Use it as a calculator too *before* you decide whether to eat something or if you are planning a meal.

ii. If you do not have access to this or another similar website tool, then use our recipes in this book with their nutritional information. You can also enter amounts in a worksheet to make your own calculations, as described below.

To calculate manually if you are not using our online automatic tracker and calculator: Enter all the foods you are eating onto the worksheet using measurements in amounts of grams. Use a nutritional guidebook which gives gram/calorie information, or go to the USDA website to get nutrient information on each of these foods. To reach the USDA website, Google "USDA Nutrient Data Laboratory", or specify the website: www.nal.usda.gov/fnic/foodcomp/search/. Whichever method you use, be sure to calculate the number of calories and appropriate number of grams of lipids, protein and carbohydrates for the serving weight you have entered for that food. For example, the information might be given for 200 grams of tomatoes but your portion is 100 grams, so you would have to reduce these numbers by half.

Keep a running total of grams of lipid, protein and carbohydrate content you are eating. Then subtotal each a couple times a day (more often in the first several days until you get a sense of size of portions), and divide each subtotal by your running total of calories to get the appropriate percentages.

After you have measured your foods during the initial two-week period you will have developed a sense for amounts, which you will have to check only once or twice a month afterward.

3. Balance

Make sure your daily food totals will fit into the protocol formula, especially (i) the **minimal oil intake of 70% of your total calories** (plus or minus 5%) **THIS IS AN ABSOLUTE MUST!!!** and (ii) 40-50 grams **protein**, which comes out to about 10-12%* of your calories, depending on calorie level, but the goal is the gram amount, not the %. The amount of **carbohydrate** intake is basically what is left over and should **never exceed 20-25%**. Less is fine, as long as you eat generous portions of greens or BalancePoint-approved vegetables that are low in calories and high in beneficial nutrients.

Quick and Easy way to do it:

i. Use an online Nutrition/Wellness Tracker as described above.

ii. **Use the Sample Days below as a template**. Usually, you can just substitute another green vegetable or tomato in a recipe and not affect the nutrient level very much so that it still stays within the BalancePoint formula. Also, you can substitute one of the meals in a Sample Day with a dish from our recipe section which matches closely in calorie count, fat percentage, and protein amount in grams.

iii. **Use snacks to adjust and balance** what you need to reach your daily total calorie goal. For example, if you find that your meals are totaling 1100 rather than 1200 calories, then add a 100-calorie evening snack; or if your meal total is reaching 1300 calories, then skip your evening snack to keep at the 1200 level.

Caution: Do not include food you are allergic to (e.g. some people have allergies to eggs or walnuts), or which your doctor has told you not to eat. For answers to some specific dietary concerns, check Frequently Asked Questions in our How I Grew Younger Guidebook: The BalancePoint

How-To and Cookbook.

Daily Calorie Targets: 1200 calories for everyone on Days 1 and 2. If you want to keep losing weight continue at 1200 calorie level Days 3-14. If you are not showing daily weight loss then reduce to 900-1000 calories. If you want to maintain or gain weight go to 1500 calories Days 3-14. CONTINUALLY MONITOR YOUR CALORIE LEVEL AND ADJUST AS NECESSARY TO MEET YOUR WEIGHT GOALS.

SAMPLE DAY - 1200 CALORIES

MEAL/SNACK	DESCRIPTION	TOTAL CALORIES	%
Pre-Breakfast	Cocoa drink *(15 grams unsweetened, non-alkalized cocoa powder and 120 grams almond milk)*	82	
Breakfast	Egg whites sautéed with 100g spinach, 26 g feta, 30 g olive oil	392	
Lunch	Binx's Stuffed Poblano *(see recipe)*	371	
Afternoon Snack	100g piece of apple	52	
Dinner	Radda Salad *(see recipe)*	302	
	Total Calories	**1,200**	**100%**
	Fat Calories		**72%**
	Protein Calories	**41 grams**	**13%**
	Carbohydrate Calories		**15%**

SAMPLE DAY - 1000 CALORIES

If, if, after Day 1 and 2, you are not losing weight on 1200 calories/day

MEAL/SNACK	DESCRIPTION	TOTAL CALORIES	%
Pre-Breakfast	Cocoa drink *(15 grams unsweetened, non-alkalized cocoa powder and 120 grams almond milk)*	82	
Breakfast	Binx's Favorite Omelet – 100 g egg whites sautéed with 30 g cilantro, 20 g garlic, 50 g Poblano chili pepper, 60g spinach, 26 g Feta, 30 g olive oil	374	
Lunch	Kale and Feta salad: 125 g shredded kale, 20 g low-fat Feta cheese, 10 g lime juice, 20 g olive oil	295	
Dinner	Asparagus Tofu Stir-Fry: 130 g asparagus, 15 g ginger, 80 g tofu, 15 g olive oil	287	
	Total Calories	**1,038**	**100%**
	Fat Calories		**67%**
	Protein Calories	**41 grams**	**15%**
	Carbohydrate Calories		**18%**

BalancePoint uses food you can buy in your neighborhood grocery store to reset your metabolism

SAMPLE DAY - 1500 CALORIES

If, after Day 1 and 2, you want to ***maintain*** or ***gain*** weight

MEAL/SNACK	DESCRIPTION	TOTAL CALORIES	%
Pre-Breakfast	Cocoa drink *(15 grams unsweetened, non-alkalized cocoa powder and 120 grams almond milk)*	82	
Breakfast	Egg whites with sautéed tomatoes *(see recipe)* Fresh apple slices *(100 grams)*	399	
Morning Snack	Walnuts (25 grams)	163	
Lunch	Asparagus in "Hollandaise" sauce *(see recipe)*, spring greens	364	
Afternoon Snack	½ Fresh peach and 7 grams almond butter	125	
Dinner	Curry kale and tofu stir-fry, Romaine lettuce	327	
Pre-Sleep	Cocoa drink	82	
	Total Calories	**1,542**	**100%**
	Fat Calories	**1,074**	**67%**
	Protein Calories	**212**	**13%**
	Carbohydrate Calories	**324**	**20%**

Yes, it can seem like boot camp for the two weeks. You are doing a lot more work than simply popping a pill three or four times a day, but that is why you are interested in doing BalancePoint—so you will not have to deal with the side effects or expense of drugs. And the protocol will start to become second nature to you so you will not need to do all the measuring after the two week initiation phase.

While BalancePoint is not a substitute for medical advice, **it may help to think of the BalancePoint protocol as a prescription. It is not a drug prescription, but a food prescription. That being said, you have to be just as exact—do not guess, do not cheat, do not do it halfway!**

EASY WAY TO GET MORE DAYS OUT OF THE SAMPLE DAYS

(without having to re-calculate your daily total nutrients!)

1. If you switch out the vegetables of a recipe for the same amount of greens and tomatoes, you will usually still be within the BalancePoint formula. For example, change the "Curry Cauliflower with Tofu Stir-fry" ingredients to Chinese broccoli with garlic and steak seasoning, or kale with chili-lime spice, or tomatoes and broccoli with lemon thyme and oregano for completely different dishes and tastes.

2. Substitute one of the meals in a Sample Day with a Chapter 17 recipe which closely matches in calorie count, fat percentage, and protein amount in grams.

Keep in mind,

- *You are not on BalancePoint* **If you are not logging and measuring** all the amounts of food you are eating (after two weeks you will start to get a learned sense of amounts). As Hippocrates stated, "Let food be your medicine," and for this medicine to work it needs to be formulated precisely every day.
- *You are not on BalancePoint* **If you are not making these VITAL calculations** every day to make sure you are fitting within the formula.: **(i)** the percentage of **lipids**, and **(ii)** minimum amounts of **protein**. Generally, watching the lipids and protein automatically takes care of the carbs, which becomes your "leftover change," so to speak. And, of course, you need to monitor the total amount of calories. Remember, we say 70% target for fat content because there is a tipping point and 60% will not work as well.
- *You are not on BalancePoint* **If you are sneaking even tiny bits of grain** into your food intake. If you are one of those very susceptible to the inflammatory effects of grain—and if you have high cholesterol you

probably are—then even "just a bite" of muffin or "taste" of pasta or serving of thickened sauce could trigger the inflammatory response we are trying to relieve your body of. And you probably did not realize you were vulnerable before experiencing the BalancePoint protocol.

- *You are not on BalancePoint* **If you are picking and choosing what parts of the protocol to follow**, even if it's "just" leaving one part out. You may believe you already know a lot about nutrition or medicine so **you feel justified in modifying the diet or trying to come up with a "better" way to do it.** You might feel there are some elements, such as type or amount of foods and calories, you want to add, delete or alter. ***Don't do it! There is a reason behind each detail of the protocol. The effectiveness of the protocol comes from being used exactly as directed***, with no deviation or changes, however little you may think they are.
- *You are not on BalancePoint* **If you try for only a few days.** The body needs to re-set itself as it opens metabolic pathways which have not been in use. Most people report finding themselves feeling more energized and "better than ever before." But there are others, especially those used to heavy carbohydrate intake, for whom this transition is not as easy. As you would expect with any new kind of regimen, some people find the first couple days uncomfortable and unsettling. We generally find that once they get through this adjustment period, these people start to feel better. Some of our biggest success stories started out with this challenge.

Consult with your doctor BEFORE you start, and if you notice any changes in your health.
Do this ESPECIALLY if you are on medications

It is a rigorous fourteen days. When you are done, though, you will be initiated into how to maintain this for life. The payoff after your two-week investment is that conditions related to chronic inflammation in your body will probably be dramatically improved. Your arthritic pain may be lessened or gone, your cholesterol level will have dropped significantly, your blood pressure and blood sugar level will show major improvements or be normalized. But now you know how to maintain your new healthy levels by letting your body take care of itself.

Measures and Conversions

1 ounce	28.4 grams
1 pound	453.6 grams
1 kilogram	1000 grams
1 milligram	.001 gram

"70-40-1200" Rule
daily goals:
70% Fats
40 grams protein
1200 calories

You can find more details, tips and shortcuts on how to do the BalancePoint protocol in the ***How I Grew Younger Guidebook: The BalancePoint How-To and Cookbook***

CHAPTER 15

What about after the 2-week Jumpstart? The BalancePoint Wellness Lifestyle

Chart 3. The Post-Jumpstart Protocol

THE POST-JUMPSTART PROTOCOL FOR OUR WELLNESS LIFESTYLE

To keep inflammation levels low and maintain healthy biomarkers

(1) When adding new foods you have not used on the 2-wk Jumpstart, such as lentils or sweet potatoes, or if you're tempted to add higher quantities of a food, such as fruit or meat, use an online Nutrition/Wellness Tracker to confirm that you are still within the important formula. "I'm eating a lot of fruit" or "not using quite as much oil" means you're off the protocol and your biomarkers will show it! It's also a good idea to keep checking once every few weeks to make sure your current diet is still compliant. (2) It is very important to continue keeping free from all grains. Don't "cheat" a little each day—our research shows that even tiny amounts of grains will bring your inflammation levels back up immediately. Once you've gone through Jumpstart, however, the recovery is easier and fairly quick. So if you take a vacation from BalancePoint go back on it completely. Remember, it is a food formula, not just guidelines. There is no "half-way" or "mostly" being on the protocol. Don't just put olive oil on everything and think you are on the protocol; in fact, never combine high-glycemic foods like grains or potatoes with high fat! If you do find yourself eating grains—and are therefore off the BalancePoint protocol—then go to a low rather than high fat diet until you go off grains again.

Fat = 70% of total calories *(min. 65%)*
Olive or canola oil, tree nuts, avocado, almond butter

40 grams Protein *(min. 35g, max. 45g)*
Egg whites, tofu, strained yogurt, feta cheese in very small quantities, nuts, greens, small portions of fish, shellfish, buffalo, grass-fed beef, pork, lamb, chicken, or duck

Chart 3. Continued

Remaining calories after reaching above fat and protein targets come from
Low Glycemic Carbohydrates *(non-starchy and non-sugar)*
(less than 80 grams/day, no more than 20-25% of total calories)
Every meal, including breakfast, should generally include uncooked weight of 150 g (min. 125 g) of a salad or greens (important to use VARIETY for different nutrients), or tomatoes and non-starchy vegetables
Handful of berries (50-60 g) and most fruit, but in small quantity, e.g. one small apple
NO fruit juice, potatoes, bananas, watermelon, carrots

NO Grains
No wheat, oats, rice, corn, barley, millet, rice starch, cornstarch—check ingredients of soups, sauces, salad dressings, sweet potato fries, soy sauce, sausages
["Gluten-free" does not mean grain-free]

Legumes OK for most people *(monitor effects) BUT watch carbohydrate level*

NO Dairy *except strained yogurt and very small quantities for seasoning only of Feta, goat and hard cheeses: Parmagiana, Romano, Manchego, aged cheddar*
Almond milk or small quantities of soy milk OK

Lots of spices for taste
Red wine, coffee, tea all OK (no beer)
Cocoa (non-alkalized, non-sweetened) (Baking cocoa) or
Dark Chocolate >85% cocoa content
Fish oil and psyllium 2Xday, multi-vitamin

Restrict and Manage Calories
Adjust as necessary according to weight goals, but keep calorie levels low. Even though you might be able to maintain weight on a higher calorie level, the health benefits you've just achieved are not preserved. These benefits are optimized by eating the minimal level of calories for maintenance

+ Exercise
+ Reduce Stress

CHAPTER 16

How to eat out—and in—BalancePoint-style

You do not have to limit yourself to cooking at home to eat BalancePoint style. You should be able to find something compliant with the protocol even if you are at Denny's or at a family reunion. You just need to approach the menu or buffet creatively and not be afraid to ask for what you want. Good humor helps! Here's a light-hearted conversation showing how Binx does it, and with more tips and recipes for home, for good measure.

Eating BalancePoint at . . .
A roadside diner?
At your mother-in-law's?
The airport?
A conference?

No Problem!

MARSHA C. IN CONVERSATION WITH BINX SELBY

Q: Now that I'm on BalancePoint, I keep wondering how you eat when you're not at home to prepare your own meals?

Binx: It's actually been no problem for me. When our bicycling group heads out on the plains, we stop in villages with very un-Boulder-like eateries. Places like, "Joe's Diner" or "Grandma's Café." I think you sort of get the hang of it. Park Café was all smokers when we used to go there but now, state law outlaws smoking inside restaurants. So, it's really quite pleasant except the place still smells like smoke but we go there anyway because it's the kind of place our group likes.

When I knew we were going to stop someplace like that, I used to bring along an apple, a handful of nuts, and a small bottle of oil oil, since I didn't expect to find anything for me.

Then one morning, when we had stopped there for brunch, down in the corner of the menu at the Park Café, I saw "Dinner salad $1.10." It was described as "mixed green." That means it's the white and not-totally-white lettuce from a head of iceberg. They get rid of any of the green stuff.

Q: They use the green to decorate the salad bar.

Binx: No, there is no salad bar at the Park Cafe. So I looked around and I noticed that someone had just gotten onion rings, served on a piece of green lettuce. I asked, "Can I have a green lettuce salad?" The waitress said, "Well we've got the regular kind of lettuce." I said, "You mean the white iceberg kind of lettuce?" She said, "That's right. That's what we've got. And we give it some carrots and cheese. We put lots of cheese in it." The carrots and cheese wouldn't work for BalancePoint. So I said, "Well, I noticed you have a garnish." She said, "What do you mean?" I said, "Well, you know, the stuff you put the onion rings on." "Oh, you mean the 'green doily'." She had some name that identified it in a completely non-vegetable way. And I said, "You know what? I want a big plate of garnish."

Q: Of green garnish!

Binx: Of green garnish. So after ordering garnish, I added, "And I want one whole tomato - sliced up. And do you have any tuna fish?" "Oh we do tuna sandwiches," she said, nodding. I thought about typical restaurant mayonnaise. It's usually made with poor quality oils and a fair amount of sugar. So I asked, "Do you have any tuna you haven't mixed with mayonnaise?" She replied, "Oh, yeah, we've got a big can." I said, "Great—I want a scoop of that on top of the garnish."

'There is no salad bar at the Park Cafe... So I said, Well, I noticed you have a garnish. She said, What do you mean?'

Q: Did you ask if it was canned in water or oil?

Binx: No, because I don't care. The oil for canned tuna is usually not the best, but they drain most of it out anyway, and I have my own olive oil along to add in. So it was fine. So then they had little bottles of hot sauces on the table—all kinds of flavors of Mexican hot sauces. This was a Hispanic area. There were four or five bottles, so I lined them up and I poured out a bit of each on different parts of my dish.

And then I remembered seeing parsley so I had them bring out some parsley. And you know, everyone around the table has got all these big pancake platters and they're looking at this thing I've got in front of me. It's a big green salad.

Remember, I also carry my little plastic bottle of olive oil and a piece of fruit. I sliced up my fruit, added it to the top of my garnish-tomato-parsley-hot sauce mixture and I had this great salad.

So, it proved to be very easy. What I do is smile and warn the waitress that I'm a troublemaker. Then they think you're really going to be a pain in the neck. And next they're astounded, "All you want is a plate of garnish?" And of course they don't know how to price it.

I got this all for $1.10. The scoop of tuna was 50 cents extra. It about broke the bank! I tell you it was about the same price as my tea.

I can order BalancePoint-compliant meals everywhere. We went to Perkins, you know, the chain? So anyway, I look at the menu. Well, it's very interesting. They have Egg Beaters that they can make for you. But I like the texture of egg whites better than Egg Beaters. So I ordered poached eggs because it's easy to take out the egg yolks. Then, when I asked what they were serving as a vegetable side, it was broccoli. So I got steamed broccoli to put around my eggs.

'Everybody at the table was looking at me enviously. This was at Perkins, and it can be anywhere.'

And it turns out that at Perkins, they make their own big dessert specials. There was a picture of one with some berries on it and a ton of confectioner's sugar. So I said, "You know what I want?" I pointed to the menu, "I want this. I want the berries just by themselves. No sugar, no cake. I'd like a cup of those berries." The waitress said, "We can do that."

When she came out with my order, she had the egg dish with broccoli on it and a great big bowl of berries. It took me two seconds to pull out the egg yolks, so that I was just eating egg whites with the broccoli, and I had my little bottle with 20 grams olive oil along to pour on them, making them even more delicious.

As for the fresh strawberries and fresh blueberries they were absolutely perfect. I asked the waitress, "Where do you get your berries?" She replied, "They come already pre-mixed. The company supplies them and we always have them fresh. We have them year-round—it's part of our standard menu. You can always get them." So, everybody at the table was looking at me enviously. This was at Perkins, and it can be anywhere.

Q: Here's my little plastic bottle of pre-measured olive oil I carry with me.

Binx: Well, that's a 60 gram-size bottle and if that's your daily allotment of olive oil, you're too low—10 or 15 grams low, even 35 grams low if you're not eating other sources of fat that day like nuts or avocados.

We recommend getting a 75-gram size bottle with a screw top, like from a camping supply store. Or if you'd prefer glass, you can get one of those glass canning jars with the screw on lids. The key is to get one that holds at least 75 grams of oil, and use it all up, every day.

People who do this are surprised at how much weight they can lose on BalancePoint with this amount of oil. It's because you need that much to keep you in lipid (fat-burning) metabolism.

Most people want to lose weight on this diet, but you don't have to. It's

'People... are surprised at how much weight they lose on BalancePoint with this [high] amount of oil.'

your choice. You still get remarkable cholesterol reduction whether you lose, gain, or maintain your weight. If you find after the initial couple days, when the body needs to lose a couple pounds to reset the metabolism, that you're still losing weight and are in the rare position of not wanting to lose more, then just add more nuts or add more oil. Or have another half an avocado.

Q: I had about 10 grams of oil today on my eggs because I figured the half an avocado I ate added fat content.

Binx: I still put oil on my half an avocado and everything else. There is definitely a tipping point, and that's why we insist you carefully measure and calculate your intake to make sure you're getting at least 65-70% or more of your calories from the oil or other sources of fat. Even 60% oil a day is too low. It's interesting that if people short themselves what they think is "only" one or two tablespoons of oil a day then the rapid reduction of cholesterol that we usually see during the two-week Jumpstart program ends up being only half what we expect.

Since I've been following the BalancePoint protocol since 2006, I'm kind of in a rhythm now where I'm pretty darn close to automatically using the right amount of oil. I can actually tell by how I feel. I know which days I'm going to lose weight and which days I'm going to gain. You get a real sense for it. A scientist who wrote about nutritional habits of primates observed that they have a real sense of what they need. They'll eat a little bit from this tree. (Gesturing) And they'll go a mile and a half over here to get a bite of that from this other tree. And then they'll go here. They have a real sense of what they need and people on our diet get it too.

People who follow our protocol also get a new sense of taste. I suspect that the traditional American diet actually dulls the taste buds. When people get away from all that and eat foods on the BalancePoint program, their taste buds come alive. Foods that they used to consider bland taste sweet, spicy, flavorful. In a salad, the green leaf lettuce starts tasting smoother, and the romaine lettuce more spicy and a little bit sweet. Green onions and red peppers start tasting amazingly sweet.

Q: Throughout the winter I like a heartier meal than a salad.

Binx: If you put the amount of oil you're supposed to put on that salad it's a very hearty meal. Drench that salad in oil.

'In a buffet line, I serve myself a big plate of greens, add the cooked vegetable. . .and a tiny bit of the meat for flavoring. There's usually a salad you can add.'

Q: Yeah, but I don't want just salad. I want something hot.

Binx: Then make a cooked vegetable. That's what I do. I'll have a big plate of chard sautéed with olive oil and garlic and ginger. Or I'll have okra or Brussels sprouts with curry.

Q: (Nodding) Like a stir fry vegetable—those kind of recipes. I even have a recipe for sweet potato and Vidalia onion roasted. It's delicious with almonds.

Binx: That's basically all right if you keep the sweet potato part to a minimum. Sweet potatoes are high in starch and especially when they're cooked, they can raise your blood sugars. That raises your insulin levels and can turn down fat-burning. Actually, that's also true if you cook a whole plate of Vidalia onions. They're on the sweet side and can get to be too much carbs if you eat too many onions.

Watch the carbohydrate calculation. It's easy to slip over that 20-25% maximum number for percentage of carbs of your daily total.

That's why we recommend something green and leafy with every meal—the greens are full of nutrients without a lot of sugars.

As for those sweet potatoes, right in the beginning during the first two weeks, keep them to a limited amount. Their glycemic index is not as high as a real potato which raises blood sugars too fast during the two weeks or after. After the first two weeks of the protocol, I still wouldn't eat sweet potatoes for every meal, but having some occasionally is fine.

By the way, something like a plate of salad greens with feta cheese, tomato, chopped up mint and olive oil is very filling. It's a great dish and really, very balanced in terms of offering adequate protein, plus if you pour on the olive oil, plenty of fat. Just because a restaurant might call this type of combination a salad, it's really more than that. It's a complete meal. It's got lots of tomatoes and wonderful mint flavor. If you can get spearmint it's really good.

Q: I'm growing spearmint. I have a ton of spearmint. So what am I going to do with it? I don't know what to do with so much of it.

Binx: I'll come and make you an awesome salad. You take a block of the low cholesterol feta. There's an organic version called Organic Valley. It's only got 10 milligrams cholesterol per pound. For 15 grams of protein, I dice up

110 grams of feta by cutting it into about ¼ inch slices and then cutting it the other way. So they're not really crumbles, but they're fairly small pieces. It's enough that the olive oil can get completely around it. And then I coarsely cut the mint. A lot of mint. At least a cupful, which amounts to roughly 60 grams. This is not a garnish. This is the salad. Get a big bunch of spearmint, not just little handful. Get the stems off, coarsely chopping it fully. Then you take a couple of big tomatoes. That's roughly 350 grams. And you dice those up into ½ inch cubes. And you put it together and toss it. Then pour 40 grams of oil over it and toss it. You can put a little French walnut oil in it for flavor if you want. So this makes two servings, and I actually like it better if it sits in the fridge for a couple hours.

Q: With that olive oil in it?

Binx: Yes, with everything mixed in. I think, somehow the mint diffuses into the olive oil and the oil diffuses into the cheese. And it's very rich. Oh, by the way, there's plenty of salt in the feta so don't put any salt on. I made the mistake of doing that once. It was very salty.

Q: Well, what about people going to conferences or workshops where the meals are all prepared? I'm going to a retreat center and they asked me if I need to have something that's gluten-free or dairy-free. I said I'm currently on a diet prohibiting grains. But what if they don't understand? Or they forget? And what if I can't tell, because they're serving something that's already mixed together?

Binx: If you tell them that you need veggies and salad, it's real easy. They almost always have things set up so that you can pick and choose. Often in a buffet line, I serve myself a big plate of greens, add the cooked vegetable—as long as it's not peas or carrots—and a tiny bit of the meat for flavoring. There's usually a salad you can add. And next to the salads, by the dressings, they often have extra virgin olive oil these days.

But just in case, I travel with my own extra virgin olive oil supply along with some lemons or limes.

And, if possible, I carry almond butter because if you need protein you can always add this to your breakfast on hard-boiled eggs (remove the yolks) or as a snack dip for fresh fruit, which you can usually find on the buffet table.

'An awesome salad… the mint diffuses into the olive oil and the oil diffuses into the cheese… very rich.'

Now, what I've said works at most conference and retreats. But I have to admit, there was one where even I came close to failing. It was one of those boot-camp Zen retreats where the whole time is spent in silence and there's only a few minutes allocated for eating. You don't say, "That's enough." It's all done in silence. So you have all of these cryptic signals for "just a little" or "more please". They're scooping into your one bowl all this stuff you can't eat. And you're not supposed to leave a crumb. So I'm trying to remember which is the signal to stop, and I'm doing the wrong thing. They think I want more.

'It's really important to carry along the oil bottle… when people stop using enough oil then the rest of the diet degenerates because the people get feeling hungry and eat the wrong things to compensate.'

After that experience, I've learned to recommend going to a retreat or business trip with a bunch of vegetables such as celery, kale and collard greens. Get some fruit like apples, pears or peaches that take a little while to ripen. Also pick up a bag of avocados. Just have that stuff so if you need it you're prepared. And then have your big bottle of olive oil with enough for the whole retreat... oh, say a half quart of olive oil, and your little bottles of, say, 75 grams for the whole day, or 25 grams for a single serving.

Before you leave home, fill your little bottles with olive oil and weigh them. Then put a mark on the side for how much will count as one serving. So if you're using your 60-gram bottle, then pour out, oh, let's say, 30 grams for breakfast, and then pour out the rest for lunchtime. Now you're at 60 grams of oil so far for the day. Before dinner, add some more oil to your bottle, say 15 grams, using the marks you've made on it to help you out. You can estimate if you have to because when you're away from home it's hard to measure.

But it's really important to carry along the oil bottle. I've found that when people stop using enough oil then the rest of the diet degenerates because the people get feeling hungry and eat the wrong things to compensate. And you're not keeping the fat and cholesterol-burners going.

I've even figured out how to do this in the airport. I've got three different small jars, each one under 3 ounces, that I fill with olive oil, and then I put them in the sealed, quart-sized plastic bag right there with my toothpaste and shaving cream, and it goes through the security posts just fine. An airport's an important place for having enough of your olive oil, just like it is at a retreat.

'Vegetable sauces for pastas... are perfecton top of salad greens or in a bowl like a stew.'

Q: That's why I started measuring it by always using my 60 gram bottle. I found I wasn't eating this much oil because you pour it on and you think you've already got a lot.

Binx: If you do a salad with the right amount of oil, when you get done you're feeling full. I do like a hot vegetable with it often. Sometimes I just put it all on the salad, sometimes on the side.

Vegetable sauces for pastas—if they haven't added sugar to them—are perfect this way. You can add them on top of salad greens if you like the sensation of a "carrier" like pasta, which adds no flavor either—just bulk. Or you can have the sauce in a bowl like a stew.

Remember to add your olive oil to it!

I also like to get some poblano peppers. They have a little bite to them. I'll dice those up and put them raw on my salad. But they're also really good cooked, one of the most flavorful things you can use. There's sort of a northwestern Spanish dish where you put some olive oil and just a little bit of water and you cook the poblanos. Sprinkle a bit of coarse salt on them. Not much if you got some kosher salt. Just a few grains on it so it's sort of like a little salt surprise. So you'll be eating it and then all of the sudden there'll be a little...

'I just asked if it was possible to get it without the breading'

Q: ...burst of salt.

Binx: Yes! Plus their spiciness. It just has a really nice flavor. So adding a lot of oil on it makes a wonderful condiment. I keep a bunch of those peppers in the fridge so that if I want some I might throw a couple of them in with the eggs in the morning. Or I love eating them as a snack.

Q: Another thing that I wanted to ask you is it seems to me that long-term we need recipes where we can make a double or triple batch, and freeze part of it. All of us are out all the time and we come home tired and hungry and that's when we're most likely to go off of a good eating plan.

Binx: That's an option, but when you can't go home there are two things that made it easier for me. One is I can eat out anywhere in the way we just talked about. The second is that more and more restaurants now are serving tasty Mediterranean-style appetizers for Happy Hour. At one restaurant I had tapas

'Mediterranean-style appetizers for Happy Hour... You can of course have that glass of wine too and still be on BalancePoint!'

or small plates. You can get things like spinach cooked in olive oil, eggplant or babganoush, mushroom caps in garlic, sautéed artichokes, tomatoes with feta. These are all done with olive oil, not butter.

One restaurant even had deep-fried tomato strip frites on the menu—I just asked if it was possible to get it without the breading and they checked with the kitchen and came back with it that way. Delicious! If the options are unusually limited, sometimes I'll just pull the breading off something.

And after the two-weeks when there's more flexibility for meat or beans, the single kabob-size portions of meat or seafood and small servings of hummus are perfect. If it's larger portions, I ask for a "doggy bag," right away, so I can slice off the portion that's too much for me, and put it out of sight and temptation. That way, I enjoy my meal and at the same time, keep it within the BalancePoint protein (40 to 50 grams of protein) or carb limits (below 20-25% of calories.) Just don't touch the pita bread, croutons or garlic toast that come with them! You can of course have that glass of wine and still be on BalancePoint! So if you have a local restaurant which serves this type of Happy Hour menu you'll find a lot of BalancePoint choices.

Q: I'm trying to find more ways to eat at home without having to go out.

Binx: Well, it's a good exercise to go out and eat because what you do is you start to look at what they've got and you 'compose.' I find it very synergistic for getting a sense of what to eat to remain on the protocol. Many people on the protocol just say they have an allergy to certain foods, and servers nod understandingly. So no grains, no sugar, no thickeners. That helps so they don't put dressing on the salad. I usually carry a whole half lemon and my olive oil with me for that.

'I've got three different small jars, each one under 3 ounces, that I fill with olive oil... put them in the sealed, quart-sized plastic bag right there with my toothpaste and shaving cream, and it goes through the security posts just fine.'

Q: The other night we were with your wife and we got lemon slices. She told us about how you always say a "wedge" because you can't squeeze a slice of lemon.

Binx: Yes, slices are good for floating in drinks but they're not good for squeezing juice on food. So I say, "A half a lemon - that's not a half a lemon made of slices." And you get the waitperson engaged. Then that's what I always do. You know, sort of make a game out of it, let them see the fun of it.

'I ask for a 'doggy bag' right away, so I can slice off the portion that's too much and put it out of sight and temptation.'

Q: Well, it makes them think.

Binx: And then they're on your side. Once that happens, then they're figuring out how to do it. Sometimes the cook comes out to check to check to see if they understood the order right. At the end I always pay my dues like to the woman who put together the plate of garnish. She brought it out sort of hesitantly, sort of like, "Did he really want this?" So I gave her a big compliment and told her what a great job she did. That tickles all the staff. Now every time I come back to one of these restaurants I'm known as the guy who eats the garnish.

Q: Your daughter loves to tell me all about her dad making a big scene. "No, no, I want the lemon like this." You can picture her face.

Binx: Yes. "Oh, Dad! It's so embarrassing!"

Q: That's what parents are for - to embarrass their children.

Binx: That's right. "Would you want me to be any different?" I ask and she replies, "Well, no, but..." You know, as long as you keep smiling and using a sense of humor the server usually tries really hard to get you what you need.

I mean, imagine how, in the middle of Wyoming at a buffalo restaurant, I see a piece of beautiful endive as a garnish on the plate going by. So guess what the waitress ends up bringing me with a big grin! By the way, after the first two weeks on BalancePoint, buffalo or grass-fed beef is one of the best meats to have if you want red meat. To keep the protein content down around 15 grams per meal, always use small portions, like two ounces of buffalo. Of course, your LDL cholesterol level will start back up again if you eat too much protein. So at the buffalo steakhouse where the smallest entrée is 14 ounces, naturally, you ask for that doggy bag, and it gives you a way to make a week's worth of delicious meals at home.

An equal part of almond butter blended with Greek yogurt is a wonderful dip for apples... totally decadent.

Speaking of home, a lot of these preparations can be kept for a period of time. Like that mint salad with the feta—feta keeps forever. And when you put feta in oil it even keeps longer. So that's one of the ones if you just keep it covered over, it really keeps well.

Q: I wasn't aware that feta was even on the first two weeks of the BalancePoint program.

Binx: You just have to make sure you get the low-fat one. It wasn't on the diet when we first created it. But because I found the low-fat version available in enough places I've decided to put it in. People like having the option to add it for taste and because many like some kind of cheese. They just have to remember to keep the amount small—only for flavor.

Q: And what about yogurt? I know you don't use the regular kind.

Binx: We use the strained, Greek-style yogurt which has just started coming out in a number of brands, like Fage, Oikos, Voskos. Some labels say, "Greek style", but actually contain cornstarch—a no-no for us—and are not strained yogurt.

Q: Are they available everywhere?

Binx: When we started back in 2006, only one place in Boulder carried Greek yogurt until so many "BalancePointers" started to go in asking for it. But now stores like Safeway and even Walmart carry one of the brands. If you're really out in a rural area, most stores are happy to place a special order for you. You can go through a lot of yogurt, not just by itself but for making things like the BalancePoint version of "Hollandaise" or "almond butter snack", so it's worth ordering a case. And you get a case price.

But there's also a very easy alternative that our friend Dee first introduced me to. Her parents have Greek and Syrian roots. They use a good quality non-fat yogurt, like Nancy's, and let it drain overnight.

All you have to do is get one of those $4 stainless steel coffee strainers at Walmart or Target, put it on top of a quart container like the plastic one regular yogurt comes in, and line it with a paper coffee filter. Set it on your counter, dump in the yogurt and let it sit there draining overnight. It's really simple.

Q: Why not drain it in cheesecloth? You want all the liquid to drain off, right?

Binx: You can use cheesecloth if you want.

Q: I'm trying to reduce the number of things in my kitchen.

Binx: The only reason to use the stainless steel ones is because they're very convenient and very clean. And you can use it over and over again. It's a permanent coffer strainer that's basket or conical-shaped.

Q: A regular strainer won't work?

Binx: A regular coffee strainer works fine.

Either way, just remember to use the paper filter. Cheesecloth is a bit coarser. Yogurt tends to get a little broken up so it's not as firm a curd. Cheesecloth was designed for this. What you're doing is trying to drain the whey off. That's what contains the hormone, insulin-like growth factor, and proteins like casein, which all tend to increase inflammation. While cheesecloth works, I find it's even better to use the real fine screens. I've tried all three and I just found that the finer screens work better. It was easier.

Doing it yourself this way makes something that tastes and has the texture of sour cream. It's non-fat. And it's more sour, which real yogurt aficionados love. You might have to develop a taste for it, especially if you're used to the regular yogurts which, if you look on the labels, are filled with sugar—and cornstarch, another no-no.

I find that once someone gets used to the deeper, more complex taste of the strained yogurt, then there's no turning back.

Both the pre-prepared Greek yogurts and the starter ones like Nancy's use a broad spectrum of very good bacteria. But it's a little different combination. The nice thing about Fage is that it's not sour, but almost a crème-fraiche.

For a snack I like to mix the yogurt with the fresh, grind-it-yourself almond butter you get at natural foods stores. So I'll take an equal part of almond butter and the yogurt and blend it together. It's a wonderful dip for apples. I mean you really feel like you're being totally decadent.

Or, you take your drained yogurt and stir olive oil into it. Then add just a little extra lime, lemon, or key lime depending on what flavor you like and you have a great "Hollandaise" for dipping artichokes, putting on eggs, using as a salad dressing.

'As long as you keep smiling and using a sense of humor the server usually tries really hard to get you what you need.'

Take artichoke hearts and chopped olives and coarsely mash together with a ton of oil and cilantro or parsley [to make] a dip for slices of fennel bulb... fantastic!

Q: I mix the yogurt with the cocoa.

Binx: Oh, do you? Now, that's interesting.

Q: And then add some nuts to it.

Binx: I've never thought of that. That's a great idea. See, we've got to share some of these recipes.

It makes me think of one of my favorite recipes. You take canned or cooked artichoke hearts and chopped olives and coarsely mash together with a ton of oil and cilantro or parsley, depending on which flavor you want to go with. It makes a dip for slices of fennel bulb. It's a fantastic recipe because it uses artichoke hearts packed in water. You can get those at Costco, six cans in a pack, something like a dollar a piece. They're real cheap. And they work great. With the olive oil, it is just totally rich and filling. Absolutely delicious.

And it's fun to pick an olive that you like the flavor of. So you go to the olive bar. This way you get to taste all of their olives, which are all on the diet. I find myself having to sample extensively before I make my choice (Laughing). But then I end up buying a whole selection because I begin to imagine other dishes I want to try them with.

It's not about deprivation or what you can't have... it becomes an opportunity... to explore and discover while enjoying some great meals.

Q: Now, see, this is what's intriguing—to introduce things that people don't normally buy or use regularly. That's what will be exciting and fun.

Binx: You're right. It's not about deprivation or what you can't have. You bring your sense of adventure and creativity to the BalancePoint diet and it becomes an opportunity. An opportunity to explore and discover while enjoying some great meals. What better way to fix your cholesterol or weight?

Summary - How to eat out BalancePoint-style

You should be able to find something compliant with BalancePoint even if you are at Grandpa Joe's or Denny's. You just need to approach the menu creatively and not be afraid to ask for what you want.

Breakfast

Most restaurants will cook egg whites only; often they are egg-beaters, which look yellow in color.

If they do not, order hard-boiled, poached or fried (hard, not over-easy) eggs so you can remove the yolks.

Ask for a side or two of vegetables. If you prefer, the veggies can instead be scrambled with the whites if they serve whites only. Almost all restaurants will have ingredients like mushrooms and tomatoes on their omelet menu; some will have avocados, artichoke hearts, and spinach; **or you might even look at their lunch menu and if you see, for example, hamburgers served with green chilies or tomatoes you can point to those vegetables for your omelet.**

Ask that they not use butter, but **fry in olive or canola oil.**

Tell them you do not want potatoes or toast/biscuit/muffin, and the like; most restaurants will substitute fruit or a salad instead.

Request a side of extra-virgin olive oil to pour over your food (breakfast is the easiest meal to get your quota of 70 grams daily or more of fats such as olive oil and we often use 50% of our oil at breakfast and then 25% at lunch and 25% at dinner); servers often bring out a blend of what they call olive oil but is really a combination of olive and canola—get them to ask if it does not look green enough for olive oil. The best bet is to carry your olive oil with you.

Believe it or not, you can develop a taste for olive oil on fruit! We know of a 4-year-old who decided to copy this practice and loves it. (His mother watched me in amazement as I poured olive oil on my fruit cup and told him about it so he decided to try it himself!)

Lunch and Dinner

Most restaurants offer salads, of course; the question will be whether you can **get dark greens, like mixed salad greens, or romaine**, or if you have to settle for iceberg, which you can dress up with toppings as described below.

A Greek salad, which seems to be appearing more and more on menus, is a good choice.

Remember to **ask for the dressing on the side; if there's sugar, balsamic vinegar or cornstarch in it, ask for extra virgin olive oil and lemon wedges instead, which is actually always the safer bet.**

When ordering a salad off the menu, tell them to hold the carrots, cheese, croutons, peas or beans, or simply remove them from your plate when it is served.

Think of your **salad greens as the base instead of pasta, rice or tortillas**; this way you can order the delicious toppings by themselves that normally form the vegetable "sauce" or filling for dishes featuring, for example, fettuccine or a burrito.

Or hunt through the menu, as explained above for breakfast, to **put together your salad toppings:**

- Nearly all diners or American-style restaurants will have **vegetable sides**, such as broccoli and cauliflower (skip the carrots), and ask if you can get them prepared without butter. Some restaurants will even sauté them in olive oil for you. Sometimes you can get sautéed spinach. Or if you see a plate go by with a garnish of curly endive ask if you can get a plate of that—"What, you want the garnish?!!!"
- In an **Italian** restaurant, look at the antipasto menu or ask if they have grilled eggplant, sun dried tomatoes, roasted peppers or other vegetables. Order a side of the meatless marinara sauce (tomato-based) and put it on your salad. This is one restaurant where you should not have to bring in your own extra-virgin olive oil, but that is not always the case.
- In a **Mexican** restaurant, look for guacamole or avocados, salsa, chili strips, tomato/onion/green pepper sauces, or burrito vegetable fillings (but watch out for the potatoes). If fajitas are on the menu, you ask for them served on lettuce or salad greens instead of rice and beans. This idea first came to us after trying a dish called "Adrienne's Special Salad," which the Home Plate Restaurant in Patagonia, Arizona created for someone on the BalancePoint protocol. It's a plate of salad greens topped with chicken fajitas, which is a delicious combo of strips of grilled chicken and sautéed red and green peppers, tomatoes and onions.

- At **fast food or airport** restaurants, you can often simply order the fillings for a sandwich, but without the bread, roll, foccacia, or flat bread. Have them put your selection on a plate of lettuce! We did that once at a panini grill at the Las Vegas airport and got a wonderful meal of grilled vegetables on salad (and quizzical looks from the young staff).

If ordering a vegetable dish at a **Chinese** restaurant, such as Chinese broccoli or greens or snow peas with mushrooms, tell them no cornstarch, no sugar, and no MSG, and of course no rice. You can order vegetables stir-fried with tofu too with the same restrictions, or ask the server/chef which dishes do not contain cornstarch or sugar; they will protest that the sauce will not be thick enough without cornstarch but just smile and say you will take it that way please. Do not use soy sauce because there is wheat in it and it is too salty. **Thai** restaurants add sugar to their sauces for American palates and many are unwilling to do otherwise, but we have come across some, like Naraya Thai in Boulder, which are happy to oblige.

If you are in a pinch you can even go to **McDonald's** and order their salad without chicken—but be aware of tantalizing aromas that might lead you in the wrong direction! You will get a bowl of greens to which you can add your own olive oil (important to get your calories and feel full) and any other vegetables (e.g. sliced peppers, which you might want to carry with you in a Baggie) or any fruit or nuts that are part of your day's allocation (which you will have to move from snack tallies).

Carry around your little bottle of olive oil and Baggies of vegetables and nuts and you will be set to dress up any meal.

Check out the **Chef Bios in Chapter 17 Recipes** to read about their restaurants and "Thumbs-up BalancePoint " dishes to get ideas of what you can order in similar restaurants in your area!

Make friends with your servers and **use good humor** about making your requests; often they will get into the challenge or fun of this unusual order. On occasion, we have had the cook, especially in diners or small cafes, come out to make sure they understand what we want so that they can get it right! (Remember to leave big tips!)

CHAPTER 17

Recipes

Guidelines for using recipes

These recipes have been carefully calculated so that you can mix and match them within the terms of the BalancePoint protocol. Each of the meals is within the 350-450 calorie specification and has an appropriate level of fat as well as protein. Without an online calculator, you will need to use judgment in balancing one recipe for use with another. For example, offset one of the higher protein ones by one of the lowest protein to make sure your daily total protein is not excessive.

Please note that simply using the recipes in this book is not the same as completely following the BalancePoint protocol. To get best results from the protocol, you must calculate your daily totals to ensure they fit into your lipid, protein, carbohydrate, and calorie targets and adapt your other food intake as necessary.

Take care to eat all the oil in a recipe. Pour any remaining oil after cooking back onto your dish, whether it is scrambled egg whites or stir-fried vegetables, because your lipid consumption compliance depends on using the whole amount. Oil is a big part of your daily calories. One tablespoon could account for as much as 1/5 of your fat content for the day. Leaving a tablespoon in the pan or on your plate everyday could reduce the beneficial changes to your cholesterol by as much as 50% at the end of the two-week program.

Simply using the recipes in this book is not the same as following the BalancePoint protocol.

BREAKFAST

EGG WHITES WITH SAUTÉED TOMATOES

- 150g tomato, cut into wedges
- 30g olive oil
- 2 egg whites
- Chopped cilantro

Optional: 30g pico de gallo (supermarket ready-made mix of chopped fresh tomato, onion, and cilantro), salsa de tomatillo, or diced green or Poblano chili pepper

- Sauté tomato wedges quickly in half the olive oil.
- Add egg whites and fold gently until cooked through. Add other half of olive oil to warm it and remove omelet to serve immediately, taking care to scoop out all the oil in the pan.
- If desired, add chopped cilantro plus one of the above salsas.

1 SERVING. 79% FAT, 8.5g PROTEIN, 325 CALORIES (9% CARBS)

Instead of tomatoes and salsa, experiment with other combos:

- Spinach, sautéed mushrooms and minced garlic
- Leftover greens like chard and collard greens with steak seasoning
- Artichoke hearts, sundried tomatoes, and Italian seasoning
- Roast tomatoes, Italian parsley, feta (10g) Middle Eastern za'atar spice
- Avocado slices with lime and pinch of chili pepper

Adrienne H. has lost 150+ pounds on BalancePoint in the past three years. This is her favorite breakfast, which she dubs,

"Israeli Breakfast"

Dice cucumbers, red peppers, tomatoes, and half an avocado and add with olive oil, salt and pepper to non-fat strained Greek yogurt. "Delicious way to start the day!" she says.

GATHERING GROUNDS "BINX SPECIAL"

Egg white omelet stuffed with feta cheese, poblano peppers, mushrooms, and spinach

When Binx would go into the Gathering Grounds Café in Patagonia, Arizona for his morning espresso, he would get former chef-owner Summer Lewton to make him a special order omelet. One day he returned to find a new menu and a dish called "Binx Special" listed. Current owners Audrey and Brandon Doles say it has become one of their most popular breakfast orders, not just for BalancePoint dieters, but also among all their customers and visiting tourists.

- 2 large egg whites*
- 50g mushrooms
- 50g Poblano pepper
- 50g spinach
- 35g crumbled low-fat Feta cheese
- 22g olive oil

Dice the pepper and slice the mushrooms. Saute the pepper and mushrooms together in half the olive oil until almost completely cooked. Add the spinach, sprinkle the inside of a lid with a few drops of water, and cover the mixture to quickly steam the spinach for about 15 seconds. Set aside and pour the egg whites into a small pan coated with other half of the oil. When the eggs have become firm on the bottom, add the mushroom-pepper-spinach mixture and the Feta. Gently fold the omelet over in half, leave on heat slightly longer to cook through, and carefully remove from pan to serve immediately, Take care to scoop out all the oil used in cooking and pour on top of omelet to serve.

*The Gathering Grounds version actually contains three egg whites, but we have reduced it to two egg whites. This way, the protein level is about half of the daily level for the BalancePoint protocol, so there is room for more protein in another meal.

1 SERVING. CALORIES: 333, PROTEIN: 18g 21%, FAT: 71%, CARB: 8%

Source: Gathering Grounds

AAA PANCAKE RECIPE

Jim F. used the BalancePoint protocol to move his triglycerides from over 700 mg/dl to the optimal level of 100 and LDL cholesterol from "too high to measure" to the ideal level of under 100 mg/dl in two weeks. After doing the 2-wk Jumpstart program, he started creating recipes such as this one as well as the two salmon meals found elsewhere in this recipe section. These pancakes are, as to be expected, of a different texture and consistency than traditional wheat-based ones and you may want to experiment yourself with ingredients, just keeping in mind the need to keep the fat% up and carb levels and calories down to stay within the BalancePoint protocol. AAA? "Almond Avocado Almond!"

- 36g almond flour (or grind almonds yourself into very fine flour)
- 66g (2 large) egg whites
- 29g avocado
- 5ml (5g) orange juice*
- ¼ tsp cinnamon

Topping:
- 5ml (5g) almond milk
- 14 g no-fat strained, Greek style yogurt
- 1 tsp cocoa

Blend almond flour with egg whites and in either a blender or food processor, add the avocado, orange juice, and cinnamon to process into a thick batter.
Makes 2 pancakes about 4 inches in diameter.
Fry over medium-low heat in a non-stick pan. Remove to plate.
Blend yogurt, almond mild and cocoa into a frothy, whipping-cream consistency for topping for the pancakes.

*BalancePoint note: We stay away from fruit juice because of the high glycemic content but this recipe calls for only 1 teaspoon to add liquid and flavor. Use a recipe like this for variety, only occasionally, because it does not supply you with the greens and veggies that an ideal BalancePoint breakfast would.

1 SERVING. CALORIES: 310, PROTEIN: 17.7g, 22%, FAT: 64%, CARB: 14%

Source: Jim F.

CHOPPED HARD-BOILED EGG WHITES COMBOS

Coarsely chop 2 hard-boiled egg whites (70g), mix with olive oil (30-35g) and try combos like one of the below:

- Salsa (50g) served on fingers of green pepper (50g)
  Calories: 327, Protein: 8.3g 11%, Fat: 82%, Carb: 8 %
- Diced tomatoes (75g), onions (25g) and cilantro (25g) and Italian seasoning
- Guacamole (25g avocado, 25g tomato, 25g onion, 15g cilantro, 10g lime juice)
- Diced red, green and yellow peppers (100g) and za'atar spice
- Green chilies, canned or sliced fresh Poblano (50g)
- Almond butter (20g)

1 SERVING

A big benefit of a high fat diet is that the oil carries spices so well and dishes become much tastier!
Be adventurous with spices and herbs to make meals interesting and give variations to basic recipes. The simple egg whites-and-tomatoes breakfast, for example, can become a different dish every day just by using Cajun, Mexican, Chinese, Greek, Indian or Moroccan flavors. Keep handy a few bottles of prepared spice mixtures, like Tuscan seasonings, chili-lime, middle eastern zata'ar, a Malaysian seasoning blend, Trader Joe's 21 Seasoning Salute, or all-purpose Montreal steak seasoning (not just for meat—try on tofu and on vegetables) to quickly transform a lunch or dinner meal into something more exotic.

Get creative with spices!

LUNCH AND DINNERS

ASPARAGUS IN "BALANCEPOINT HOLLANDAISE" SAUCE

- 175g fresh asparagus
- 25g olive oil
- 25g strained, Greek-style non-fat yogurt
- 15g lemon juice
- 125g mixed greens
- 10g roasted unsalted almonds

Sauté asparagus in 5g olive oil until barely tender.
Blend the remaining 20g olive oil with the yogurt and lemon juice to make Hollandaise sauce.
Arrange asparagus on a bed of salad greens, drizzle sauce on top and garnish with the almonds.

1 SERVING. CALORIES: 351, PROTEIN: 10.1g 11%, FAT: 74%, CARB: 15%

Source: How I Grew Younger Guidebook: The BalancePoint How-To and Cookbook by Binx Selby, Linda Jade Fong and Robert Kerr ©2012

TOMATO, FETA AND MINT SALAD

We discovered this salad at a café on a bicycle trip in southern France about 15 years ago. After coming home, we recreated the recipe and have enjoyed this version ever since.

- 350g tomatoes
- 40g olive oil (or 30g olive oil and 10g French walnut oil)
- 110g reduced fat Feta
- 60 g spearmint or mint (at least 1 cupful)

Cut the block of Feta into ¼ inch-slices and then make ¼-inch slices the other way, so that you are getting 1/4 inch cubes. Cut the stems off the spearmint and chop coarsely. Dice the tomatoes into ½-inch cubes. Put the Feta cubes, spearmint and tomato cubes into a bowl and toss. Pour the oil over the mixture and toss again. Let sit in refrigerator if possible for a couple hours before serving.

2 SERVINGS. CALORIES: 657 (329 FOR 1 SERVING), PROTEIN: 27.6g (13.8 FOR 1 SERVING), FAT 73%, CARB: 11%

Source: Binx Selby

CURRY CAULIFLOWER AND TOFU STIR-FRY

This is a basic stir-fry recipe for use with any vegetables, such as tomatoes, mustard greens, bok choy, broccoli, or kale. Adjust cooking times to prevent overcooking. Vary the seasonings to give a different flavor and version of the dish. You might try bok choy with ginger, garlic and wheat-free soy sauce, or kale with chili-lime spice, or tomatoes and broccoli with lemon thyme and oregano.

- 5g grated ginger
- 4-6g (1-2 tsp) minced garlic
- Dash of curry powder (or more to your taste!)
- 25g olive oil
- 50g diced firm tofu
- 180g cauliflower sliced ¼ inch thick
- 60g (¼ cup) chicken or vegetable broth
- Accompaniment—125g Romaine lettuce

Sauté the ginger and garlic in half the olive oil over medium heat for one or two minutes until soft but not colored. Add the tofu and a dash of curry, and stir-fry gently for two minutes (or longer if you like it crisper.) Add the sliced cauliflower, toss quickly to coat in oil, and add half of the chicken or vegetable broth. Cover and cook for 2 minutes. Remove cover. When liquid has evaporated, stir-fry everything quickly to pick up seasonings from the pan and add the remaining broth. Cook uncovered until almost all of the liquid evaporates, stirring occasionally.
Mix in the other half of the olive oil. Serve warm on bed of Romaine lettuce.

1 SERVING. 375 CALORIES, 14.2g 14% PROTEIN, 67% FAT, 18% CARBS

GINGER CHARD WITH TOMATOES

This dish, created by Binx, was voted one of the favorite dishes at our BalancePoint gourmet tasting! Make sure the dish is served while still hot.

- 20g fresh, unpeeled ginger, (1 piece 2 inches long—quite a large amount, don't scrimp!)
- 25g olive oil
- 80g fresh chard
- 100g tomatoes (Roma tomatoes work the best but all kinds work, cut in ½ inch pieces)

Peel the ginger and thinly slice, cut slices into toothpick-size pieces. Cook ginger on very low heat in 10g of olive oil for 2 minutes. Set aside. Heat 10g of olive oil in a stock pot or other large pot using highest heat available. When oil is starting to ripple from the heat, before it starts to smoke, put in chard. Add the cooked ginger and continue cooking, stirring often until the chard starts to wilt. As soon as the ginger is added to the chard, heat remaining 5g of olive oil in a second large pot using high heat. Add tomatoes to this second pot and cook for 2 minutes, then add to chard mixture. Salt to taste. Serve immediately while still hot over bed of romaine lettuce or salad greens.

1 SERVING. CALORIES: 270, FAT 81%, PROTEIN: 3g 4%, CARB: 15%

Source: How I Grew Younger Guidebook: The BalancePoint How-To and Cookbook by Binx Selby, Linda Jade Fong and Robert Kerr ©2012

CLASSIC GREEK SALAD

- 50g tomatoes
- 50g cucumbers
- 25g Kalamata olives
- 25g onion
- 25g olive oil
- 50g low-fat, low-cholesterol feta
- Salt
- Oregano

Cut the tomatoes into wedges and slice or cube the cucumbers.
Break feta into bite-sized pieces. Cut olives into halves. Slice onion thinly.

Mix olive oil, salt, and oregano and toss all ingredients together. This is the classic Greek salad, but for variety try adding sun-dried tomatoes and artichoke hearts.

1 SERVING. CALORIES: 385, PROTEIN: 11.6g 12%, FAT 80%, CARB: 8%

Source: How I Grew Younger Guidebook: The BalancePoint How-To and Cookbook by Binx Selby, Linda Jade Fong and Robert Kerr ©2012

BINX'S STUFFED POBLANO PEPPER

This dish is always a big hit among friends who enjoy the rich, sometimes hot, taste sensations of poblano peppers. The recipe also works well using the milder regular green, red or yellow peppers.

- 100g (1 medium to large size) poblano chili pepper
- 30g fresh cilantro leaves (stems removed*)
- 60g crumbled low fat Feta
- 25g olive oil

Wash Poblano, cut around stem and pull out stem with seeds. Mix crumbled feta with cilantro leaves, and stuff mixture into the pepper. Press finger into stuffing to create a "well". Pour olive oil into this well. Place pepper in uncoated stainless steel or cast-iron skillet. Set the skillet under preheated broiler and cook pepper until it is well blistered and partially blackened (about three minutes). Turn pepper over and broil other side until it blisters and partially blackens.

WHAT IS A POBLANO?

Poblanos are mild, heart-shaped chili peppers commonly used in Southwestern and Mexican cooking. They are large and have thick walls, which make them ideal for stuffing. Chile rellenos are often made with poblanos, as are many sauces and salsas. The "heat" is found mainly in the seeds and membranes, so you may want to remove the seeds and veins before cooking (wash hands carefully with soap afterward and don't rub your eyes!) Even so, poblanos can range from mild to hot and it is generally impossible to predict, but that is part of the rich flavor! For a milder version of any of our recipes calling for a poblanos, substitute a regular green, red or yellow pepper.

Put on serving plate and pour all the oil and cooking juice from the skillet over the pepper—eat all the oil since it is included in the fat% calculation and it is very tasty!

*To remove stems: Grab a stem of cilantro and pull it through the thumb and finger of your other hand so that the leaves get stripped off. If the stem breaks off so that only the upper, tender part of the stem remains with the leaves, go ahead and keep it along with the leaves.

1 SERVING. CALORIES: 371.4, PROTEIN: 14g 14%, FAT: 78%, CARB: 8%
Source: Binx Selby

QUICK WATERCRESS AND TOFU SOUP

- 350 ml (350 grams or 3/4 pint) low-salt chicken, beef or vegetable stock (check label to make sure it's wheat-free)
- 125g watercress, torn into small pieces (or substitute spinach or Romaine lettuce)
- 30g soft or medium tofu, cut into½ inch cubes
- 1 spring onion (shallot), chopped
- 20 g olive oil
- Salt
- Freshly ground black pepper

Bring the stock to a boil in a saucepan. Add the spinach and tofu. (If you are using soft tofu, handle carefully so that it doesn't break up too much.) Bring back to a boil, then add the olive oil, spring onion and salt and pepper to taste. Simmer for about ten minutes; do not overcook or the vegetable will lose its green color and the bean curd will become tough. Serve hot.

1 SERVING. CALORIES: 347, PROTEIN: 15g 17%, FAT: 65%, CARB: 18%

WHY WE USE GRAMS IN OUR RECIPES

Grams are a convenient and accurate way to measure all types of food. You can be more precise with weight than with volume, such as tablespoons or cups. Now that low-cost electronic kitchen scales are readily available, it is easy to measure in grams. Olive oil is especially important to measure because it makes up such a big portion of your calories, and being a tablespoon off for the day could be 20% of your fat calories. This means you might not reach the tipping point of going into lipid metabolism if you do not get enough of your calories from fat. Will you always have to measure everything you eat? No. You will be surprised at how you quickly begin to develop a sense for how much 25g of olive oil or 150g of salad greens is.

ROASTED—OR EVEN CRISPY—BRUSSELS SPROUTS

(Or asparagus, red peppers, kale, zucchini, cauliflower!)

Cut Brussels sprouts vertically into ¼-inch slices and toss with olive oil, salt, pepper, and minced garlic. Lay out on a foiled cookie sheet in a 500° oven. Put onto middle shelf of oven and roast to your preferred level of doneness, about 7-10 minutes. We prefer to leave the vegetables roasting until charred and crispy. This is a way to solve the craving some people have for something crunchy to munch on—either as a side dish or snack (instead of taco chips!) Experiment with different veggies! Spices like a little curry, Middle Eastern za'atar, Eastern European Vegetal, or cumin could be interesting too...

TOASTED SESAME SPINACH SALAD

- 150g spinach, small leafed preferable (or 100g spinach and 50g arugula)
- 30g fresh cilantro
- 15g (1 ½ Tbsp) sesame seeds
- 2g (1/2 tsp) sesame oil
- 1 to 2 small Mexican (key) limes
- 50g silken, lite tofu
- 22g olive oil

Toast the sesame seeds on baking pan in preheated 400° oven. Watch carefully and as soon as they start to turn color, remove immediately and shake onto a piece of tin foil to cool. Remove stems from cilantro. Toss the cilantro leaves and spinach together. Add the sesame seeds. Squeeze juice from the limes and toss. Dribble the sesame oil over the salad. Cut tofu into 1 inch square, ¼ inch thick pieces, add to salad. Toss well so that the tofu picks up flavors of the other ingredients. Add the olive oil, toss and serve.

1 SERVING. CALORIES: 357 PROTEIN: 10.6g 11% FAT: 77% CARB: 12%

Source: Binx Selby. Either reduced fat tofu or silk tofu are preferable for the texture for this salad.

Source: How I Grew Younger Guidebook: The BalancePoint How-To and Cookbook by Binx Selby, Linda Jade Fong and Robert Kerr ©2012

CHILLED AVOCADO, LIME AND CILANTRO SOUP

- 340g ripe avocados
- 70g mild onion, chopped
- 1 garlic clove, crushed
- 2 Tbsp chopped fresh cilantro
- 1 Tbsp chopped fresh mint
- 30g (2 Tbsp) lime juice
- 700g (700 ml) vegetable stock
- 1 Tbsp light soy sauce (wheat-free)

To garnish:
- 15g Greek-style yogurt
- 1 Tbsp finely chopped cilantro
- 10g (2 tsp) lime juice
- Fine shreds of lime rind
- 1 Tbsp vinegar
- Salt and pepper

Halve, pit, and scoop out the flesh from the avocados. Place in a blender or food processor with the onion, garlic, cilantro, mint, lime juice, and about half the stock and process until completely smooth.

Add the remaining stock, vinegar and soy sauce and blend again to mix well. Taste and adjust seasoning if necessary with salt and pepper or with a little extra lime juice if necessary. Cover and chill in the refrigerator until needed.

To make the lime and cilantro cream garnish, mix together the yogurt, cilantro and lime juice. Spoon into the soup just before serving and sprinkle with lime rind.

2 SERVINGS. CALORIES: 664, PROTEIN: 10.2g 7%, FAT: 68%, CARB: 31%

BalancePoint note: This recipe has a higher carbohydrate % than our usual recipes. Be sure to balance it with much lower carb recipes so that your total carb intake for the day is no more than 20-25% or your calories.

Source: Adapted from Cookshelf Thai (Paragon, 2003)

3-NATION SALAD

We call this recipe "3-Nation Salad" because it combines Chinese lettuce, Italian sundried tomatoes and Moroccan preserved lemons. That's what happened to catch Linda's eye looking in the refrigerator one day, and voila, a crisp and colorful salad with unique bites of flavor! You can buy the preserved lemons in a Middle Eastern grocery, or you can easily make your own with directions we give you on this page.

- 125g Chinese lettuce (also known as "siu choy" or "Napa cabbage")
- 25g sundried tomatoes (julienned)
- 20g olive oil
- 20g Moroccan preserved lemons

Cut the head of lettuce in half lengthwise and then cut cross-wise into no wider than ½- inch slices for the portion size you wish. Slice the preserved lemons into thin ¼-inch strips. Toss the lettuce,

PRESERVED LEMONS—THE SECRET INGREDIENT!

I lived in Morocco for six months when I was a student. I discovered preserved lemons, the magical element which gives a slightly tart and salty, and intensely lemony, flavor to the fabled cuisine of Morocco. You can buy the preserved lemons in a Middle Eastern grocery, or order them on Amazon, or make them yourself. Here's how: Slice the lemons as if you were going to quarter them, but don't cut all the way through the base. Then generously shake Kosher salt over them and press them into a large jar. .Add water to ensure that the lemons are covered with brine. If you don't see undissolved salt crystals, then you need to add more salt to make sure preserved lemons, julienned sundried tomatoes, and olive oil together, and you have created a one-of-a-kind salad in less than 5 minutes!

1 SERVING.
CALORIES: 261
PROTEIN: 3g 4%
FAT: 77%, CARB: 19%

Source: Linda Jade Fong

the liquid is saturated. Don't worry about having too much salt, because you can't—extra salt crystals will stay in the solution and you will rinse off any excess salt anyway. Reverse the jar periodically (make sure you have a tight lid!) and let the jar sit for 30 days. Then you are ready to use the lemons! Pull out of the brine as needed, rinse off, and slice or dice to add as your secret ingredient for salads, fish, meats and vegetable dishes! - Binx Selby

---

STIR-FRIED LETTUCE WITH SOY SAUCE

- 1 head Romaine lettuce
- 25g olive oil
- 1 garlic clove, minced
- 1 teaspoon (5 ml) pale dry sherry
- 1½ teaspoons (7 ml) wheat-free soy sauce (check ingredient label)

Separate the lettuce into leaves and break into 2 inch pieces. Put lettuce into salad spinner and blot any remaining water on leaves with paper towel. Heat half the oil in a pan and add the garlic and sherry, and then the lettuce leaves. Cover and cook for 1 minute. Arrange on a serving dish and pour all oil from the pan plus the remaining half of the olive oil over the lettuce. Sprinkle the soy sauce on top of the lettuce and serve hot as a main dish, or cold as a salad.
Note: Broccoli or Chinese cabbage (bok choy) may be used in place of lettuce.

CALORIES: 340, PROTEIN: 8.8g 10% , FAT: 66%, CARB: 24%

CHRIS MUELLER

Chef/Owner

Red Lion Restaurant, Boulder, Colorado

People still talk about the formal birthday dinner that Chris gave his mother in his large restaurant in Boulder when she was visiting from Germany. After the entrée, he brought to her table a young man who, Chris explained, wanted to sing for the former opera singer. No sooner had the man gotten through a few off-key lines of Happy Birthday than the music suddenly changed. Frau Mueller's expression changed from polite nodding to horrified shock as the "singer" flung off his trench coat. Her son, the prominent restaurateur, had brought in a male stripper for her 80th birthday treat.

Chris's mother was not only an opera singer, but also a professional cook in their native Germany. So six-year-old Chris was pressed into early service making cookies for guests one day when there was no cake in the house. In 1961, Chris came to the U.S., where he re-connected with a girl he used to play with in the sandbox back in Germany. Heidi was now a very American, tall blonde. They fell in love, got married, and together bought an almost 100-year-old restaurant, which had been operating since 1870. Named the Red Lion, it was beautifully situated in the mountains just outside Boulder, on the banks of the creek rushing through Boulder Canyon.

Under the smiling eyes of Chris and Heidi, and now their daughter Tina, the Red Lion has been one of Boulder's top tourist destinations and favorite wedding spots for over 40 years. Locals bring visitors to enjoy a taste of the West, where wild game entrees enliven the continental menu, rustic stone walls surround fireplaces, and a softly lit outdoor dining pavilion down over the creek offers an uniquely Boulder experience.

It's a perfect spot for BalancePoint diners to celebrate graduating from the two-week Jumpstart program. This is when meat in small, four-ounce portions can be re-introduced into the diet. You might select from game such as elk or boar on the menu, or you may opt to indulge in one of the half a dozen cuts of buffalo, always a two-thumbs-up meat option for the BalancePoint Wellness Lifestyle. The 8-16oz cuts are large enough for two to four BalancePoint portions, so you have plenty to take home to freeze for a later meal, or to enjoy the next day sliced up atop a salad!

RED LION KALE WITH PEARS

German-born Chris Mueller explains that, before the days of greenhouses, kale was the vegetable that was available fresh all winter in Northern Europe. In fact, European gourmets would not eat kale until the first frost. Even now in Colorado, Chris puts kale in the freezer for an hour before making his favorite Northern European recipe, "Kale with Pears."

- 150g kale, deveined so that you are using the leafy, soft part of the kale
- ¼ medium-sized onion
- ½ small pear
- ¼ tsp nutmeg
- ¼ tsp salt
- 2g olive oil
- 80g (⅓ cup) chicken or beef bouillon

Chop kale into ¼ inch pieces (like parsley). Chop onion. Heat oil, not too hot. Cook onions until shiny with a little brown glazing. Add salt and nutmeg. Add chicken or beef bouillon to onions and olive oil. Add kale and simmer for 40 minutes. Add pears, pitted and quartered. Cook for 5 minutes. (For BalancePoint, we do not like to cook fruit more than necessary to keep glycemic load as low as possible.)

1 SERVING. CALORIES: 358, PROTEIN: 6.6g 7%, FAT: 62%, CARB: 31%

BalancePoint note: This recipe has a higher carbohydrate % than our usual recipes. Be sure to balance it with much lower carb recipes so that your total carb intake for the day is no more than 20-25% or your calories.

Source:* *Chris Mueller

MATTHEW JANSEN

Chef/Owner

Mateo Restaurant Provencal and Radda Trattoria
Boulder, Colorado

Nationally-recognized chef Matthew Jansen started off his life in Colorado-poster-boy fashion. He grew up in Boulder, graduated with a degree in Journalism from the University of Colorado, and was a member of the National Ski Team. Touring with the ski team, he got a taste of fine dining in ski resorts around the world. He was primed for this because he had grown up as a "surrogate son" of the Laudisio family, who brought sophisticated Italian dining to Boulder. Besides working at their restaurant and learning recipes handed down from Grandma Laudisio, he and Tavio Laudisio spent four autumns working in the grape harvests and cellars of great wine-makers in Italy and France. This led to Matthew's earning the sommelier certificate from the Court of Master Sommeliers of London. Matthew then went on work in leading roles in acclaimed restaurants such as Aqua, Aqua Bellagio, and Charles Nob Hill in San Francisco and Las Vegas.

Matthew is now chef-owner of Boulder's Mateo Provencal Dining and Radda Trattoria, both highly recognized dining venues in a city which is second only to New York City for restaurants per capita. Like many Mediterranean-style restaurants, these two offer dishes already perfect for a Balance Point meal, such as Nocciole Miste— roasted mixed nuts—and Verdure alla Griglia — grilled escarole, fresh herbs, agrumato (an olive oil often infused with lemon zest.) Others are easy to adapt, such as the Ravioli al Tonno, which is braised tuna, cauliflower, treviso (a red form of endive), toasted almonds, and Tuscan olive oil. This is normally served in a raviolo pasta, but Matthew's chef team does a version as a topping for fresh romaine or grilled kale.

Matthew's success has been lauded locally and nationally: Bon Appétit selected Radda as one of the Top Ten New Restaurants in the country in 2007. Try his recipes and you will see for yourself how simplicity can lead to sophisticated gastronomical tastes you might not have ever associated with a "diet" before. Your dinner guests will be as impressed. After all, Bon Appetit certainly was!

Calorie restriction without suffering

RADDA INSALATA

The menu changes regularly at Radda Trattoria, a neighborhood restaurant inspired by the cuisine and culture of Tuscany, Italy. But you can always be sure to find this salad on the menu. It's been popular ever since the restaurant opened five years ago, and once you try this recipe you'll see why.

- 125g Belgian endive
  [halve the head of endive and finely chop length-wise before measuring]
- 2g white truffle oil
- 18g extra virgin olive oil
- 10g fresh squeezed lemon juice
- 10g hazelnuts [toasted and crumbled]
- 10g shaved parmigiano-reggiano (45g)
- 1g Italian parsley [finely chopped] (5g)

Combine olive oil and lemon juice (slowly add to form an emulsion). Lightly toss endive, crumbled hazelnuts, parsley and lightly dress with olive oil and lemon dressing. Salt and pepper to taste. Arrange salad on chilled plate. Top with shaved parmesan. Finish with light drizzle of truffle oil.

1 SERVING. CALORIES: 302, PROTEIN: 6.7g 9%, FAT: 83%, CARB: 8%

Source: Matthew Jansen, Radda Trattoria

RAPINI DALLA GRIGLIA – GRILLED RAPINI

(also known as broccoli rabe or choy sum)

Share chef Matthew Jansen's secret on how to make delicious grilled vegetables. He suggests, "This recipe works very well with kale, swiss chard and braising greens mix (we do not blanch the chard and braising mix; rather, sauté in a hot cast iron skillet.)" We think you'd also find success using Matthew's recipe with even more vegetables, like Chinese broccoli (similar, but not as bitter as rapini), broccoli, cauliflower, or asparagus.

- 150g rapini
- 12g extra virgin olive oil (48g)
- 12g parmigiano-raggiano [shaved] (45g)
- ½ cup vegetable stock
- 1 cup water
- ⅛ tsp red chili flakes
- 1 tsp garlic [minced]
- 20g lemon [juiced]

Boil water and vegetable stock. "Blanch" rapini in boiling liquid for two minutes. Place rapini in ice water bath. Remove rapini and place in colander to remove excess moisture. Drizzle very small amount of olive oil on rapini. Salt and pepper to taste. Finish on wood burning grill [turning once until hot but not over blackened] or conventional gas grill. Combine remaining olive oil, garlic, lemon and chili flakes. Lightly toss rapini in dressing. Arrange rapini on plate to serve.

1 SERVING. CALORIES: 238, PROTEIN: 12.4g 20%, FAT: 62%, CARB: 18%

Source: Matthew Jansen, Radda Trattoria

SNACK IDEAS

Kale Chips

Brush fresh kale leaves with olive oil on both sides. Arrange in one layer on a cookie sheet and lightly sprinkle with salt. Bake at 350°until the leaves are dried out and crunchy-crisp.

Source: Maryanne Bruno

Apple slices

dipped in almond butter

Berries

mixed with roasted walnuts

Dark chocolate >85% cocoa

(Wellness Lifestyle post 2-week Jumpstart)

TIPO DI ZUCCA (BAKED SQUASH)

Note from Chef Matthew: This squash recipe works very well for a variety of winter squash (cooking times may vary slightly.) This is a dish that we enjoy during the fall and winter months. The wood oven imparts a wonderful smokiness to a variety of foods and also has fantastic, intense heat. But conventional ovens are perfectly adequate in the absence of a wood burning oven. Buon appetito!

- ½ acorn squash (halve the squash lengthwise and clean)
- 20g extra virgin olive oil
- ½ Tbsp cinnamon
- 1 sprig fresh thyme

Rub squash lightly with olive oil. Place squash face down in roasting pan and bake for 45 minutes [450°]. Slice each half in approximately six slices. Dust with cinnamon. Salt and pepper to taste. Lightly toss with sauté pan in wood burning oven until caramelized [725°] or conventional oven [450°]. Arrange squash on one large or four small plates. Finish with fresh thyme leaves and olive oil drizzle. Serves four.

4 SERVING. CALORIES: 1028 (257 FOR 1 SERVING), PROTEIN: 7.6g (1.9g FOR 1 SERVING), 3%, FAT: 64%, CARB: 33%

***Source:** Matthew Jansen, Radda Trattoria*

BalancePoint note: This recipe has a higher carbohydrate % than our usual recipes. Be sure to balance it with much lower carb recipes so that your total carb intake for the day is no more than 20-25% or your calories.

MARCO MONNANI

Chef/Owner

Bacco Trattoria, Boulder, Colorado

Parma Trattoria Mozzarella Bar, Louisville, Colorado

When you think "diet" you do not normally think of "Duck breast with Dried Cherries" or "Fennel with Anchovy and Pernod." But those were just some of the twenty dishes chef Marco Monnani created for our BalancePoint Tasting Party in 2007 to introduce the gourmet possibilities of our protocol.

Marco was born and raised in Italy, where his grandmother would store plum tomatoes in five to six hundred beer bottles for making sauce in the winter. The sauce might be used to top a huge cornmeal polenta made on a wooden table and then covered with grilled vegetables. Everyone in the family would sit down together to eat this truly "one-dish" meal, and this is a dish that Marco easily adapted to the BalancePoint protocol, by leaving out the polenta, keeping the delicious sauce and vegetables, and making it even more mouth-watering by increasing the amount of olive oil. Inspired by his grandmother, Marco started cooking as a teenager. He then studied at a cooking school in Verona before working on the Princess Cruise Line for two years. The rigor of preparing three meals a day and different cuisines every night introduced him to an abundance of techniques.

His experience led to chef positions in England, New York, Switzerland, and Las Vegas. An avid skier, he came to Boulder, Colorado and fell in love with the area. He has been a chef-owner of several leading local restaurants, most recently Bacco Trattoria, and has surprised many a visiting European to find such authentic northern Italian cuisine in the American west!

Marco continually creates new recipes, like adding wasabi to portobello mushrooms, which reflect his international experience and have proved easily adaptable to our BalancePoint protocol. Whatever the dish, Marco says, "My recipes are simple—four or five ingredients—but they match well."

MARCO'S SALMON

Chef Marco Monnani likes the delicate flavor of North American salmon and how it matches well with caramelized onions.

- 22g olive oil
- 15g red onion
- 14g sugar (optional)
- 1 tsp red wine vinegar
- 120g salmon
- 1 lime

Put olive oil in sauté pan and heat for about 2 minutes. Using medium to high heat, sear the salmon on each side for about 1 and a half minutes. Add red onions, sugar and a teaspoon of red wine vinegar. Squeeze a lime over it and cook for about 3 more minutes.

*We do not use sugar in the BalancePoint protocol, but Chef Monnani likes to use sugar to caramelize the onions. We suggest trying the recipe without the sugar first and seeing if you find that the onions get enough of a caramelized effect for you without the sugar. Also, we recommend using a half-portion of this recipe served with a salad or greens.

1 SERVING. CALORIES: 475, PROTEIN: 24.2g, 20%, FAT: 65%, CARB: 14%

MARCO'S FENNEL WITH ANCHOVY AND PERNOD

This is a traditional recipe from Rome where the distinctive ingredients of anchovy, garlic, fresh mint and extra virgin olive oil combine to give the fennel a wonderful flavor.

- 2oz olive oil
- 7g mint
- 4g anchovy
- 7g garlic
- 112g fennel
- 1 tsp pernod

Cut the fennel in two parts. Put in boiling water for about 5 minutes.
Put olive oil in sauté pan. Add anchovy, fennel, garlic. Sauté on medium to high heat for about two minutes. Deglaze the pan with the teaspoon of pernod. Add the fresh mint and the rest of the olive oil and it is ready to eat.

2 SERVINGS. CALORIES: 580, PROTEIN: 2.6g, 2%, FAT: 86%, CARB: 7%

***Source for both on this page:** Marco Monnani*

TSUKASA HIBINO

Chef/Owner

Sachi Sushi, Niwot, Colorado

Tsukasa Hibino never imagined that he would one day open a sushi restaurant in Colorado. He graduated with a degree in landscape design in 1979 in his native Japan, and decided he would like to go to Brazil. But he spoke only Japanese, so he thought he would head to Brazil via Los Angeles, where he could learn English. He ended up spending four years in L.A. He then thought he should look for a small city to see more of America.

He picked Boulder. At a local seafood restaurant, he met another Japanese man and fellow Mah-jongg player who persuaded Tsukasa to try his hand at making sushi. They worked together for three years before embarking in 1987 to open a sushi restaurant, Sushi Tora, on Boulder's Pearl Street Mall. It quickly drew in Japanese clientele driving from as far as Denver, thirty miles away, for its authentic cuisine. From that success, Tsukasa went on his own in 2006 to open a small Sushi bar named Sachi Sushi, a hidden treasure hidden inside the back corner of a village market in Niwot, Colorado. So now Denver customers and restaurant reviewers drive even further to seek out Tsukasa.

Wearing his trademark baseball cap and wide grin, Tsukasa can often be found running the tiny restaurant himself, as he makes dishes to order while cheerfully chatting up customers. He likes to bring in non-traditional elements, especially American, to his sushi. His BLT sushi is a big hit and we couldn't resist tasting it by scraping away the rice! His cooked fish specials, like black cod, salmon and other fatty fish, get BalancePoint endorsement when you ask for it with salad instead of rice.

When asked to adapt some recipes for BalancePoint, Tsukasa laughed and said he had never used olive oil or left out rice for making sushi before—this would be a challenge. The results are delicious, as you can taste for yourself!

SALMON SAUTE

- 114g slice of salmon (preferably wild)
- 14ml (14g) wheat-free soy sauce
- Salt and pepper
- 30ml (30g) wine vinegar
- 15g olive oil

On the sliced salmon, spread salt and pepper and some of the oil. Put the rest of the oil in frying pan, add the salmon, then cook with small fire with lid. Add the wine vinegar and soy sauce. Transfer to plate with all the oil.

1 SERVING. CALORIES: 314, PROTEIN: 26.2g 34%, FAT 64%, CARB: 1%

SALMON SAUTÉ WITH AVOCADO SALAD FOR JUMPSTART MID-POINT

Half way through the 2-week Jumpstart program, the BalancePoint protocol allows a one-time serving of salmon to add variety—a sort of treat, if you will. (After the 2 weeks, you can begin to add fish or meat in small enough amounts to keep within daily total protein of 35-40 g.) Here's how to take a recipe, like "Salmon Sauté" above, and lower the portion of salmon but add avocado and salad greens or Romaine lettuce so that you can get a meal which fits into the BalancePoint protocol for calories, protein and fat amounts.

- 60g wild salmon
- 7ml (7g) wheat-free soy sauce
- 150g Romaine lettuce or salad greens
- Salt and pepper
- 20g olive oil
- 15ml (15g) wine vinegar
- 34g avocado slices

Prepare salmon as in "Salmon Sauté" recipe above, using 15 g of the olive oil. Place salmon in the middle of a plate of Romaine lettuce or salad greens. Arrange avocado slices around the edge of the plate. Drizzle all he pan oil over the fish and the remaining 5 g of olive oil over the lettuce.

1 SERVING. CALORIES: 354, PROTEIN: 16.3g 18%, FAT: 73%, CARB: 9%

Source for both on this page: Tsukasa Hibino

RATNA SHRESTHA

Chef/Owner

Nepal Cuisine, in Boulder

The ingredients list for the recipes Ratna Shrestha has prepared for BalancePoint might at first glance seem long. But look again and you will see that most of them are spices, often a dozen or so in a dish. They all contribute to the complex, richly layered flavors of Himalayan cooking. In addition to adding flavor, Ratna says there is a Nepalese tradition of using spices for their health-giving properties. So turmeric might be sprinkled in to boost memory and reduce inflammation, or fenugreek seeds might be tossed in to help with conditions like diabetes and high blood pressure.

Ratna was raised in the restaurant business and learned the art of spices from her parents, who had a restaurant for 30 years in Kathmandu. The small country of Nepal boasts eight of the world's ten highest mountains, including Mount Everest. But it does not boast the best educational opportunities for women. So Ratna and her husband Machendra brought their two young daughters to the U.S. in the early 1990's. It was a good move. Their older daughter is a nurse pursuing medicine and the younger is a journalism graduate.

Ratna continued her love of cooking in her new country and in 2007, she and Machendra opened their second restaurant, Nepal Cuisine, in Boulder, Colorado. . As in most Indian and Nepalese restaurants, customers can count on BalancePoint-friendly vegetable dishes, such as cauliflower or spinach, as well as meat dishes where you can pick small BalancePoint-size portions.

Ratna says she never follows recipes, but instead picks something from the market and sees what comes to mind. That is how a dish using summer squash, pork spareribs and tomato gets inspired (recipe in *How I Grew Younger Guidebook: The BalancePoint How-To and Cookbook.*) Her customers always delight in their discovery of new tastes,, such as okra or mustard greens in oil-rich, spicy sauces. Indeed, you will see from the recipes in this book that Ratna's creations are unlike any you'd find in other Indo-Himalayan restaurants.

There's another reason, though, why Ratna and Machenra draw an intensely loyal customer base. Ratna pours love not only into her cooking, but also into her customers. You are greeted like old friends and, if you've been sick, might be given a bowl of the best chicken soup in town to take home!

NEPAL CUISINE TOMATO AND TOFU ACHAR

This is an exquisite dish, one of the best tomato and tofu recipes we've ever tried—in any cuisine! Chef Ratna Shrestha was inspired by a dish from her hometown of Kathmandu, where they grill tomatoes on a fire and grind them together with green chili, garlic and cilantro, to create this variation with tofu for American kitchens.

- 225g Tofu cut into bite size cube pieces
- 105g olive or mustard seed oil
- 672g chopped onion
- 720g chopped tomatoes
- ½ Tbsp – minced garlic
- ½ Tbsp – grated ginger
- ¼ tsp fenugreek seeds
- ⅓ tsp tumeric powder
- ½ Tbsp salt
- ½ Tbsp cumin powder
- ⅓ tsp coriander powder
- ⅓ tsp chili powder
- 5g (⅓ cup) cilantro

Using medium heat, heat oil in a non-stick pan. Fry tofu pieces until they turn a light golden brown color. Carefully remove from heat and set aside. Add fenugreek seeds in the same heated oil. When the fenugreek seeds reach a dark brown color, add garlic, ginger, turmeric powder and stir. Once garlic turns light brown, add remaining ingredients and mix well. Cook for 15 minutes, stirring occasionally. Lastly add fried tofu and chopped cilantro. Serve on top of Romaine lettuce if you wish.

5 SERVINGS. CALORIES: 1585 (317 FOR 1 SERVING), PROTEIN: 42g (8g FOR 1 SERVING) 10%, FAT: 64%, CARB: 26%

Source: Ratna Shrestha

SPICES AND MEDICINAL PROPERTIES

by

RATNA SHRESTHA

Ajwain seeds

Used as a digestive aid.

Turmeric powder

Has anti-inflammatory properties, has been found to be helpful in fighting Alzheimer's, rheumatoid arthritis, cancer, and cystic fibrosis.

Cumin

aids in digestion, and helps relieve cramps and pain in abdomen.

Cardamom

known to help with pain and gas.

Fenugreek seeds

useful for diabetes and high blood pressure

MUSTARD GREENS WITH SOYBEANS

Did you know that Edamame beans, so common at Japanese restaurants and backstage as healthy snacks for celebrities these days, are soybeans? For this recipe, you can buy Edamame beans from the supermarket and remove the beans from the pods, like shelling peas. Or, you can go to an Asian grocery and buy already skinned soybeans! Chef Ratna Shrestha suggests that you try this recipe with other greens as well, such as bok choy, rapini, or Chinese broccoli, to substitute for the mustard greens.

- 224g washed and cut mustard greens
- 100g soybeans
- 70g olive, mustard seed or canola oil
- 1 Tbsp cumin powder
- ¼ tsp fenugreek seeds
- ⅓ tsp coriander powder
- ⅓ tsp red crushed pepper
- 1½ Tbsp chopped garlic (14g)
- 60g chopped tomato
- Salt

Heat vegetable oil in a saucepan and fry fenugreek seeds until dark brown. Add chopped garlic, and sauté until golden brown. Add soybeans and fry for about 4 or 5 minutes. Add mustard green, remaining spices and stir. Cook for 5 minutes.
Garnish with chopped tomatoes and serve on Romaine lettuce leaves.

3 SERVINGS. CALORIES: 880 (293 FOR 1 SERVING), PROTEIN: 24g (8g FOR 1 SERVING), FAT: 80%, CARB: 12%

Source: Ratna Shrestha

BADRIA BEDRI
Women, Infant and Children Nutrition Expert
Nogales, Arizona

Badria Bedri's great-grandfather in Sudan had nine daughters and no school that would take them in. Only males were allowed upper education. So he started a women's school in his own house. The small town did not like the idea and kicked them out. He found a piece of land for his campus and put the ownership in the name of the Sudanese people, not the government or the family. It became the first women's university in Sudan and the only one of its kind in Africa and the Middle East.

Fifty years later, that university sent his great-granddaughter Badria to the U.S., to Iowa State. The goal was for Badria to learn about nutrition, so that she could become a health educator back in Sudan. But it did not turn out that way. As Badria was finishing her B.S. and M.A. degrees in Nutrition, she met future family physician Joel Block. Badria and Joel got married in Sudan then settled in Nogales, Arizona on the Mexican border, where they raised their two daughters now off at college. Badria works as a nutritionist for WIC, a federally-funded nutritional program for women, infants and children in low-income families.

Her recipes for BalancePoint give hints of not only her Sudanese background, but also the Italian culinary skills of her mother, who grew up in an Ethiopian orphanage run by Italian nuns. When BalancePoint offers "fusion" recipes, we mean it!

BADRIA'S OKRA

Sudan native, Badri Bedri, adapted this from a traditional recipe of her homeland. If the recipe looks Middle Eastern to you, it's not surprising. Many Sudanese dishes reflect the Lebanese, Turkish and Egyptian cuisine of people who have populated the country.

- 180g young fresh okra or frozen
- 25 olive oil
- 35g onion, chopped
- 1-2 gloves of garlic, chopped
- ¼ tsp. coriander
- Salt and pepper
- 75g tomato sauce (unsalted)
- 1½ tsp. lime or lemon juice

Clean okra with slightly damp cloth. Cut off the stems. Sauté in 1/3 of the oil until lightly brown. Set aside, taking care to keep all the oil you used to cook with. Add another ⅓ of the oil to the same pan and sauté the chopped onion, garlic and seasonings, till the onion is slightly yellow/ transparent. Add the okra sauté for a minute then add the tomato sauce and enough water to barely cover the okra. Add the remaining ⅓ of the oil and cook on medium heat for 20-25 minutes, stirring every now and then. Add the lemon or lime juice and let it cook for 5 minutes more.

Note: if frozen okra is used omit the sautéing of the okra. After the 2-week Jumpstart, you may add meat, such as a small portion of ground buffalo or grass-fed beef, to this dish. The meat is browned first, then you add the onion step.

1 SERVING. CALORIES: 310, PROTEIN: 5.1g 6%, FAT: 69%, CARB: 25%

Source: Badria Bedri

PARSLEY AND TOMATO SALAD

An easy and very refreshing salad!

- 1 bunch Parsley, preferably the Italian flat-leafed kind, but the curly type works well too
- 170 Grape tomatoes (or Roma tomatoes) chopped very small
- Juice of 1 Mexican lime (key lime)
- Olive oil
- ¼ tsp white vinegar
- Dash of Allspice
- Salt and pepper

Trim the parsley keeping a little bit of the stems with the leaves. Chop very coarsely. Put into small bowl and toss with the chopped tomatoes, olive oil, lime juice, vinegar and allspice. If you wish, add one chopped green onion.

1 SERVING. CALORIES: 213, PROTEIN: 1.8g 3%, FAT: 82%, CARB: 15%

Source: Badria Bedri

ROASTED EGGPLANT WITH MIXED VEGGIES

- 915g (2 med.) eggplant
- 120g green pepper seeded and diced
- 120g red pepper seeded and diced
- 150g onion sliced
- 1 clove of garlic chopped
- 63g olive oil
- 2 tablespoon red wine vinegar or any other non-Balsamic vinegar
- Salt and pepper
- Cumin (optional)

Wash all veggies before cutting. Peel the eggplant, remove as much of the seeds as you can, and then cube and salt the eggplant for about ½ hour. Pat eggplant dry with a paper towel. Combine all veggies in a baking dish, drizzle using up all the olive oil over them, add salt and pepper, stir well. Bake at 400 degree for 45 minutes, stirring once in a while. Add vinegar and cumin and toss.

3 SERVINGS. CALORIES: 912 (304 FOR 1 SERVING), PROTEIN: 13.5g (4.5G FOR 1 SERVING), FAT: 61%, CARB: 33%

*Source: Badria Bedri. Adapted from **Don't Play With Your Food, Spring and Summer Cook Book** by the Arizona Nutrition Network.*

EGGPLANT WITH TOMATO SAUCE

Badria Bedri tasted an eggplant and tomato sauce dish she really liked in a Persian restaurant. She could never find it again—so she recreated it herself!

- 2 med. eggplants sliced about 1 inch thick, spread on a sheet, sprinkled with salt left for ½-1 hour and atted dry before frying.
- 60g onion diced
- 2-3 cloves of garlic, chopped
- 100g Olive oil
- 300g of crushed or diced tomatoes
- Salt and pepper
- 1 Tbsp tomato paste
- 10 leaves Basil or ¼ tsp cumin

Fry the slices of eggplant in the oil until lightly browned. Remove the eggplant slices to another plate, but do not blot the oil from them, and do not drain away oil from pan.
Cook the onion and garlic till transparent in the remaining oil in the pan. Add crushed tomatoes. If diced tomatoes are used blend them a bit in a blender before using. Add salt and pepper. Add tomato paste. Let onion and tomato cook on medium heat and stir occasionally for 20 minutes. Add the fried eggplant to the tomato sauce and cook for 10 minutes and add the herb of your choice.

4 SERVINGS. CALORIES: 1304 (326 FOR 1 SERVING), PROTEIN: 18.8g (4.7 FOR 1 SERVING), FAT: 66%, CARB: 28%

Source: Badria Bedri

NIKOS AND MARIA PSILAKIS

Who better than the co-founder of the Greek Academy of Taste to provide us with tantalizing recipes? And even better when the recipes come from the island of Crete, whose people have shown the best cardiovascular health in the world, and whose traditional diet rich in olive oil and greens is closely aligned to BalancePoint?

Nikos Psilakis founded the Academy to educate the world as well as younger generations on the island about the Cretan diet. It has been part of his mission, along with wife Maria, to document and help preserve rituals of the land which, in ancient days, boasted the Minoan civilization and legends of the Labyrinth, and, more recently, a health-giving lifestyle seen in 115-year-old shepherds in the mountains. For over 20 years, Nikos and Maria have travelled across the peaks, valleys and coasts of Crete to collect recipes and study the food culture of villages and farms.

Nikos is an award-winning journalist, author, historian, photographer, and poet. His talents combined with Maria's skills as a cook, writer and educator have resulted in some of the most exquisite and fascinating cookbooks you will ever come across. *Cretan Cooking, The Secret of good Health—Olive Oil, and Herbs in Cooking* are a delight to the taste buds and to the eyes, with every page lavishly illustrated with Nikos's photos. The biggest bonus for us is that 80-90% of the recipes are BalancePoint-perfect or easily adaptable!

To meet this remarkable couple is to be embraced by warm smiles that start with their eyes. It is not surprising that Nikos has written children's books as well as a book about Cretan monasteries and sacred trees. There is more to their recipes than just expertise in the health aspects of the Cretan diet, and perhaps you will feel it too as you try them!

YOGURT DIP WITH DILL

- 300g non-fat strained yogurt
- 1 Tbsp dried dill
- 1 mashed clove garlic
- Salt and pepper
- 27g olive oil
- 15g (1 Tbsp) lemon juice

In a deep bowl, beat yogurt with dill, garlic, salt and pepper. Add olive oil and lemon juice. Beat until well mixed. Keep refrigerated. Goes well with vegetables and green salads.

2 SERVINGS. CALORIES: 413 (207 FOR 1 SERVING), PROTEIN: 27.4g (13.7G FOR 1 SERVING) 26%, FAT: 59%, CARB: 15%

YOGURT DIP WITH PARSLEY

- 300 g non-fat strained yogurt
- 2 Tbsp dried parsley
- 70g onion, grated
- Salt and pepper
- 27g olive oil
- 15g (1 Tbsp) lemon juice

Beat yogurt with onion, parsley, salt and pepper. Continue to beat the mixture, adding olive oil and lemon juice until well mixed. Store in the fridge.

2 SERVINGS. CALORIES: 438 (219 FOR 1 SERVING), PROTEIN: 28g (14G FOR 1 SERVING) 25%, FAT: 55%, CARB: 19%

AVOCADO DIP

- 272g avocados
- ½ tsp salt
- ½ tsp pepper
- 70g onion, grated
- 5g (2 Tbsp) finely chopped parsley
- 25g olive oil

Peel avocado, remove the pit and then mash it in a deep bowl. Add the other ingredients and beat with a whisk until creamy. Garnish with parsley and keep the dip in the fridge. Use it on its own to dip appetizers and small vegetable pieces or on meat or fish or even on salads.

2 SERVINGS. CALORIES: 708 (354 FOR 1 SERVING), PROTEIN: 6.4g (3.2G FOR 1 SERVING) 6%, FAT: 80%, CARB: 16%

Source for all 3 Dip Recipes: Adapted from ***Nikos and Maria Psilakis, Olive Oil,*** *used with permission.*

MEAL IDEAS FROM JIM F.

(700+ TRIGLYCERIDES DOWN TO ~100 IN 2 WEEKS)

Jim F. used the BalancePoint protocol to move his triglycerides from over 700 mg/dl to the optimal level of 100 and LDL cholesterol from "too high to measure" to the ideal level of under 100 mg/dl in two weeks. He is an avid F. fisherman and here are two salmon meals he created:

POACHED SALMON WITH BOK CHOY AND GINGER SWEET POTATOES

Put orange slices in pan and fill pan with water just enough to cover the orange slices. Place salmon on top (don't cover with water), add combination of olive oil, black pepper, white pepper, multi-colored pepper, Club House lemon spice mixture and/or other herb seasoning. Cover pan with lid and steam 10 min/inch of thickness of salmon.

Sauté baby bok choy with a few ¼-inch slices of yellow peppers (for color) in olive oil with a touch of wheat-free soy sauce.

Cook small portion of sweet potato (be mindful not to exceed carb level of protocol) in microwave, and then mash with olive oil and ginger.

SALMON WITH BLUEBERRIES, FENNEL AND SQUASH, GREEK SALAD

Grill or fry salmon no more than 10 minutes total per inch (5 minutes if only ½-inch thick.) Mix wheat-free soy sauce and water (4 parts water to 1 part soy sauce), ¼ tsp honey, and oil. When honey is dissolved, add scant handful of blueberries. Drizzle sauce over salmon.

Greek salad of chopped orange peppers, Roma tomatoes, yellow peppers, red onion, cucumber and fresh basil.

BAKED ACORN SQUASH AND FENNEL

- Baked acorn squash and fennel
- 30g acorn squash
- 30g apples
- 30g of fennel bulb
- 15g walnuts or almonds for texture.
- 20g white wine
- 20g olive oil
- Spices: fresh rosemary and/or lemon thyme and or greek oregano (whatever you have around!) Sage is too strong. Salt and pepper to taste. Cube acorn squash and apples. Cut fennel.in ¼ inch slices. Mix together with walnuts, white wine, olive oil and spices. Bake covered until desired softness is achieved

1 SERVING. CALORIES: 329, PROTEIN: 3g 4%, FAT 82%, CARB 15%

MEAL IDEA FROM SUSAN B.

(ARTERIAL AGE DOWN FROM 100-YR-OLD TO 45-YR-OLD IN 2 WEEKS)

70-year-old Susan B. dropped her LDL cholesterol from 160 to 73 mg/dl, a drop of 87 points, in two weeks on BalancePoint. In addition, her arteries, which measured as stiff as a 100-year-old's before BalancePoint, regained the flexibility of a 45-year-old in these same fourteen days.

"Tonight my 'entree' was sautéing bite-size pieces of asparagus in olive oil until nearly done, then adding sun-dried tomatoes in their oil, and cooking for a bit. When I dished it up I added Trader Joe's feta made from sheep's milk in small chunks. This was accompanied by a big salad with Sunflower Seed Dressing. It was very tasty and satisfying."

SUNFLOWER SEED SALAD DRESSING

- ½ Cup sunflower seeds
- ⅓ Cup apple cider vinegar
- ¼ Cup wheat-free tamari
- 1 Cup extra virgin olive oil (or canola)
- ⅓ Cup cold water

Blend all in blender until seeds are pulverized and no longer recognizable, but do not over-blend. Add another 1/3 Cup cold water and stir to blend. This keeps well in refrigerator. It will separate, but blends back together easily.

AFTER THE 2-WEEK JUMPSTART

FOR THE WELLNESS LIFESTYLE

These recipes are for the BalancePoint Wellness Lifestyle, when you can start to add small, no more than approximately 4 ounces, of protein sources such as fish, buffalo, grass-fed beef. Just be sure that your total protein for the day still stays in the 35-40 gram range. So if you are eating meat, for example, do not also eat additional sources of protein such as eggs and yogurt the same day. The best way to add meat is to think of using it more as flavoring, rather than as an entrée. With that approach, you are using only tiny amounts, not even necessarily the full serving size of the recipes below—and you can buy the best quality with such small portions!

DUCK WITH DRIED CHERRIES

Chef Marco Monnani explains that in traditional haute cuisine, duck is usually cooked with a sweet sauce, such as A l' orange or Sweet and Sour. Since the BalancePoint protocol shies away from using sugar, Marco instead uses a tiny amount of dried cherries to add a creative and delicious twist.

- 2oz olive oil
- 4g dried cherries
- 140g duck breast
- 7g fresh sage

Put olive oil in sauté pan and heat for about 2 minutes. Using medium to high heat, sear the duck breast for two minutes on each side. Add dried cherries and sage and cook for about 4 more minutes.

2 SERVINGS. CALORIES: 658 (329 FOR 1 SERVING), PROTEIN: 35.2g (17.6 G FOR 1 SERVING), FAT: 77%, CARB: 2%

Source: Marco Monnani

MARCO'S FILET MIGNON

This dish, along with the Duck with Dried Cherries, were two of the biggest hits at the BalancePoint gourmet tasting which Chef Marco Monnani presided over in 2007. This delectable cut of meat is also very low in saturated fat and cholesterol, so it works well as an occasional BalancePoint treat. However, ounce per ounce, meat is also very high in protein, so Marco pays special attention in this BalancePoint version of Filet Mignon to make a satisfying meal with a smaller portion of meat.

- 20g olive oil
- 64g crimini mushrooms
- 140g grass-fed beef or buffalo tenderloin
- 7g rosemary

Put olive oil in sauté pan and heat for about 2 minutes. Sear the meat on medium to high heat for two minutes on each side. Add mushrooms and let them cook with the meat for about 4 more minutes. Sprinkle fresh rosemary on top and serve.

1 SERVING (OR 2 SERVINGS IF YOU USE THE DUCK AS A TOPPING FOR A SALAD OR BED OF GREENS TO WHICH YOU ADD A LITTLE MORE OIL—A WONDERFUL MEAL!). CALORIES: 410, PROTEIN: 31.2g, FAT: 67%, CARB: 3%

Source: Marco Monnani

SEA BASS WITH PURSLANE

Purslane is a summer wild green that is starting to become the "new Arugula" in trendy restaurants and greenmarkets. It is a highly prized salad green in most of Europe and is often served chopped with garlic, lemon juice, olive oil and salt in yogurt in countries such as Crete and Turkey. Purslane's small, fleshy leaves, flowers and stems have a lemony, slightly salty flavor that adds a distinctive note to salads. Purslane is loaded with Omega-3 fatty acids, and perhaps that is why it was used by the ancient Greeks as a dietary remedy for inflammatory conditions.

- 1 kilo sea bass (1000g)
- 1 finely chopped onion
- 1 clove of finely chopped garlic
- ½ kilo crushed tomatoes (500g)
- 1 kilo roughly chopped purslane (1000g)
- 160g olive oil
- Salt and pepper

Scrape, wash and gut the fish. Cut into 8 slices and sauté in 60 g of the oil, turning them over to brown evenly. Take the fish out and put the onion in the skillet. Brown the onion for a few minutes and add the garlic, the tomato, the purslane, the remaining 100 g of oil, and 1 cup water. Cook for 10 minutes and place the fish again in the skillet, over the purslane. Salt and pepper. Cook for another 10 minutes. Serve each slice of fish surrounded by a ring of purslane on the plate. Serves 8.

8 servings. Calories: 2,680 (335 for 1 serving), Fat: 60%,
Protein: 200g (25g for 1 serving), 30%, Carb: 10%

Source: Adapted from recipe of Maria and Nikos Psilakis, Cretan Cooking

TOFU, TOMATO AND BASIL

- 182g tomatoes
- 70g bacon
- 5ml wine vinegar (5 g)
- Little bit of basil
- 225g silk tofu
- ½ green onion
- 2.5 ml wheat-free soy sauce (2.5g)
- 10g red pepper
- Little bit of dried bonito
- Black pepper

Slice tomato into ½ inch slices. Put 1-pound weight on tofu for 30 minutes, then wipe the water away from around the tofu. Then slice into ½ inch slices.
Slice the bacon thinly. Then very thinly slice the red pepper and green onion. Mix in a bowl with wine vinegar, soy sauce, olive oil and add a dash of black pepper.

Put on a plate with the sliced tomato, sliced tofu and basil. Spread with dried bonito top with oil/vinegar sauce.

2 SERVINGS. CALORIES: 500 (250 FOR 1 SERVING), PROTEIN: 25.7g (13G FOR 1 SERVING), FAT: 68%, CARB: 11%

Source: Tsukasa Hibino

Other new BalancePoint Wellness Lifestyle recipes such as "Tuna Carpaccio" by Tsukasa Hibino or "Squash with Spare Ribs" by Ratna Shrestha can be found in the *How I Grew Younger Guidebook: The BalancePoint How-To and Cookbook and Cookbook.*

SEE THE *HOW I GREW YOUNGER GUIDEBOOK: THE BALANCEPOINT HOW-TO & COOKBOOK* FOR:

- MORE "HOW TO" INSTRUCTIONS FOR DOING THE BALANCEPOINT PROTOCOL
- "SHORTCUTS AND TIPS"
- MORE DETAILS ON WEIGHT MANAGEMENT

OVER 100 NEW RECIPES! INCLUDING

No-grain Waffles
Mexican Spinach Salad
Sweet and Sour Shrimp
Fish in Parchment Paper Wraps
Grilled Eggplant with Tahini
Squash with Spareribs
and
Fennel Salad with Grapefruit and Pine Nuts

APPENDIX 1

Before/After 2-week Changes in Cholesterols, Triglycerides, and Arterial Stiffness for BalancePoint Study Participants

Measure	Beginning Group Mean	End Group Mean	Mean Difference	Significance	Risk Assessment
N=25					
Total Cholesterol (mg/dl)	222.480	166.360	-56.120	p<0.001	desirable <200
Triglycerides (mg/dl)	114.000	84.200	-29.800	p=0.004	normal <150
HDL (mg/dl)	58.200	59.560	1.360	p=0.46	high >60
LDL (mg/dl)	142.160	90.080	-52.080	p<0.001	optimal <100
VLDL (mg/dl)	25.932	19.916	-6.016	p=0.002	8< normal <25
Non-HDL (mg/dl)	164.280	106.800	-57.480	p<0.001	<130
LDL/HDL Ratio	2.472	1.528	-0.944	p<0.001	Low risk <3.3
N=15					
Radial Systolic Pressure (mmHg)	134.867	127.067	-7.800	p=0.05	
Radial Diastolic Pressure (mmHg)	83.133	79.533	-3.600	p=0.098	
Aortic Systolic Pressure (mmHg)	126.467	114.933	-11.533	p=0.004	104<normal<128
Aortic Diastolic Pressure (mmHg)	84.133	80.333	-3.800	p=0.089	
Aortic Pulse Pressure (mmHg)	42.333	34.600	-7.733	p=0.001	29< normal <15
Aortic Augmentation Pressure (mmHg)	14.133	7.267	-6.867	p<0.001	4< normal <15
Aortic Augmentation Index (%)	31.667	19.467	-12.200	p<0.001	
Aortic Augmentation Index @ HR 75 (%)	26.300	17.000	-9.300	p<0.001	9< normal <32
Arterial Age Equivalency using Aortic Augmentation Pressure (yr)	69.200	50.400	-18.800	p=0.001	
N=18 Participants electing wt loss*					
Weight (lbs)	169.517	161.650	-7.867	P<0.001	
Body Mass Index	26.197	24.979	-1.218	p<0.001	normal <24.9

**Not all study participants wanted to lose weight, and weight loss is not necessary to achieve the other desired outcomes.*

The results shown in this table demonstrate that all measures changed in a healthy direction during the two weeks on dietary program, and with respect to the lipid profile (top seven rows); all but one, HDL, were statistically significant. Average lipid profile improvements were dramatic: total cholesterol lowered by 25 percent, LDL by almost 37 percent. Perhaps the most helpful results were that non-HDL cholesterol was decreased by 35 percent and the LDL/HDL ratio dropped by 38.2 percent.

The above table shows the results of a study of 25 BalancePoint participants in a study named, "Dietary Protocol for a Rapid Reduction of Risk Levels of Cholesterols, Triglycerides, and Arterial Stiffness: A Before/After Study of a Pilot Dietary Program" (R. Williams, B. Selby, J. O'Hearne, R. Selby, R. Kerr).

The "Significance" column in the table shows that even though the sample size is small, the amount and consistency of change give statistical significance indicating confidence in the results. The "p" means "percentage" so, for example, if p = .001 then the probability of that result happening by chance is 1/10 of 1%.

APPENDIX 2

The Effect of the BalancePoint Protocol on Arterial Stiffness in 2 Weeks

Sphygmographic charts for 65-year-old male in study, "Dietary Protocol for a Rapid Reduction of Risk Levels of Cholesterols,Triglycerides, and Arterial Stiffness: A Before/After Study of a Pilot Dietary Program"
(See Appendix 1)

HEMODYNAMIC PARAMETERS BEFORE PROTOCOL

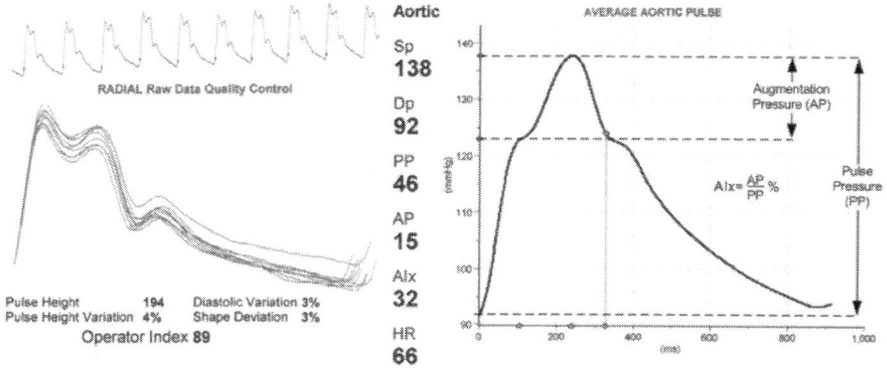

HEMODYNAMIC PARAMETERS AFTER PROTOCOL

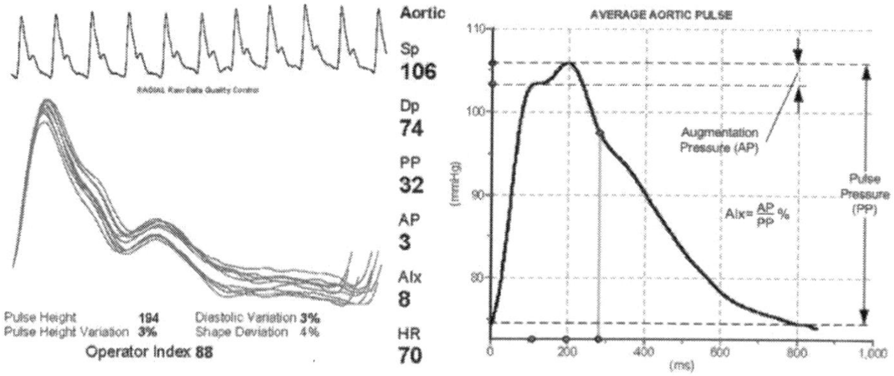

The first graph, "Before protocol", shows the higher internal aortic pressure that results from stiffer arteries: aortic augmentation pressure ("AP") of 15 mmHg and total aortic systolic pressure ("Sp") of 138 mmHg. The second chart, "After protocol", shows the aortic pressure after 2 weeks on the BalancePoint dietary protocol: aortic augmentation pressure reduced from 15 to 3 mmHg and total aortic systolic pressure reduced from 138 to 106 mmHg. These decreases are a result of reducing arterial stiffness, which is a risk indicator for stroke. It appears that the BalancePoint protocol lowered inflammation levels to produce these reductions. When these aortic augmentation pressure readings are charted on an FDA-approved database seen below, the age equivalency of these readings drops from what would be considered normal for a 65-year-old (this exact correlation of arterial age to chronological age is coincidental) to that of a 20-year-old. This is one example from our study, and results vary from person to person. **The average change in relative age equivalency was a reduction of 18.8 years of age** *(c.f. Appendix 1).*

ARTERIAL AGE EQUIVALENCY BEFORE AND AFTER PROTOCOL

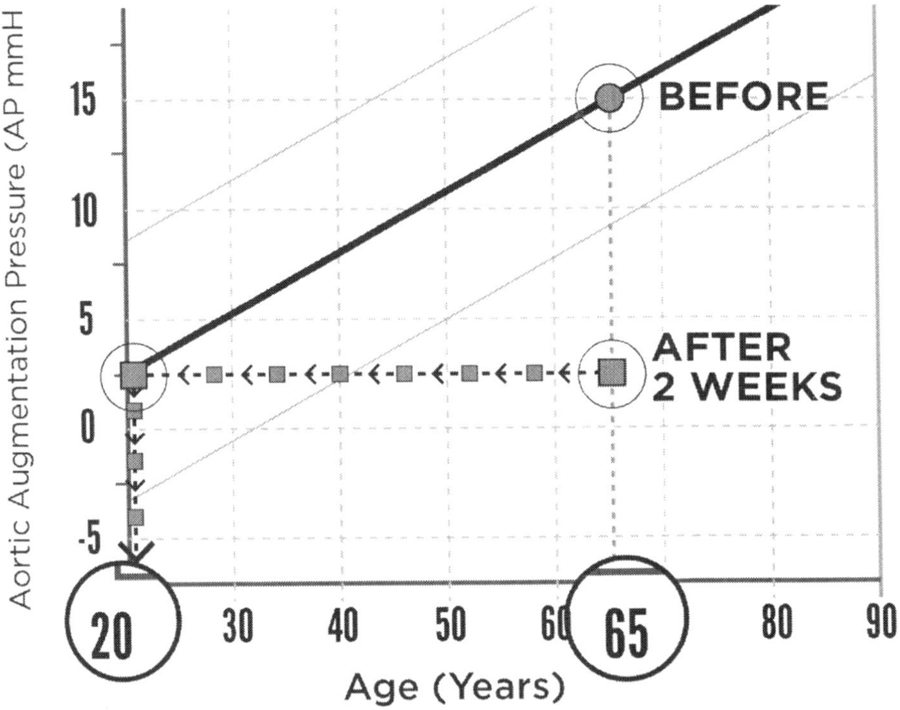

INDEX

P

R

S

T

U

V

W

Y

ABOUT THE AUTHORS

Binx Selby is an inventor whose biochemistry research goes back to his days as a student, when his undergraduate work earned him an early invitation to join Sigma Xi, the scientific and engineering research society. He went on to start over a dozen companies around his diverse inventions. These included the NBI word processor, which was one of the first personal computers, and the PureCycle on-site total water recycling and purification system, which was featured in media as diverse as Walter Cronkite's science show on TV to *National Geographic* and *R&D Magazine*'s Top 100. His latest invention is an anti-inflammatory dietary protocol which re-balances the biochemistry in our body to reverse and prevent the onset of age-related diseases, and which has produced supporting test results since 2006. When not doing research for his new Lifestyle for Health Research Institute, Binx can be found riding his bike, singing in choirs, or doing comedy with a local theater group.

Linda Jade Fong received national and international awards for her work as an editor before starting ventures such as Technology Information Corporation and Caravan International Publishing. Most recently, she has co-founded with Binx Selby the non-profit Lifestyle for Health Research Institute to study how to achieve robust longevity, and, true to its spirit, has recently made her debut in an over-age jazz dance troupe.

26463316R00115

Made in the USA
Lexington, KY
02 October 2013